THE
*S*ECRETS
OF
AIKIDŌ

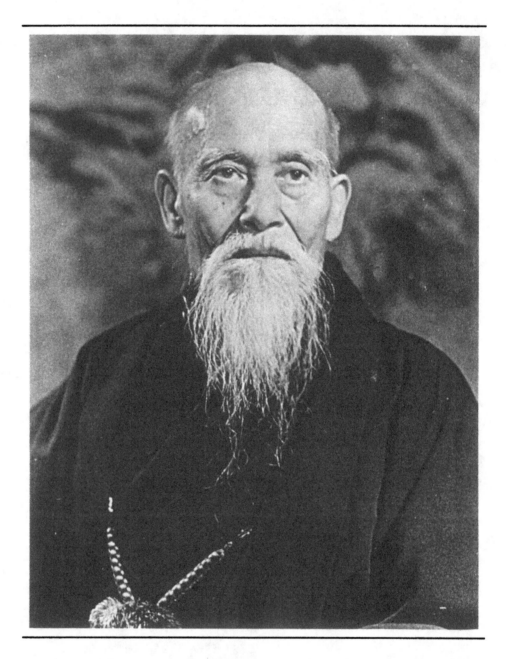

Morihei Ueshiba (1883–1969), the Founder of Aikidō: "If you have life in you, you have access to the secrets of the ages, for the truth of the universe resides in each and every human being."

THE
SECRETS
OF
AIKIDŌ

JOHN STEVENS

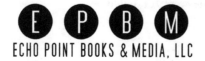

ECHO POINT BOOKS & MEDIA, LLC

Published by Echo Point Books & Media
Brattleboro, Vermont
www.EchoPointBooks.com

The Secrets of Aikido
ISBN: 978-1-62654-325-6 (paperback)

Cover photo courtesy of the author

Interior design by Ruth Kolbert

Cover design by Adrienne Núñez
Editorial and proofreading assistance by Ian Straus,
Echo Point Books & Media

Dedicated to
Rinjirō Shirata Sensei (1912–1993),
who openly taught me the secrets of Aikidō

C O N T E N T S

Preface ix

P A R T O N E
STUDY OF THE WAY
THE MYSTERIES OF AIKIDŌ

AIKIDŌ: *The Way of Harmony* 3

KOTOTAMA: *The Language of the Gods* 15

KAMI: *The Divine Alchemy of Fire and Water* 27

KI: *Universal Energy* 36

KOKYŪ: *The Breath of Life* 44

CHINKON-KISHIN: *Calming the Spirit, Returning to the Source* 53

MISOGI: *Purification of Body and Mind* 62

REI: *Gratitude and Respect* 70

SANGEN: *Triangle, Circle, Square* 77

MA-AI: *The Right Place* 81

TENGU: *The Master Teachers* 87

RYŪ-Ō: *The Dragon King* 95

MASAKATSU AGATSU KATSUHAYABI: *True Victory* 104

PART TWO
WALKING THE PATH
THE PRACTICE OF AIKIDŌ

SHUGYŌ: *Constant Training*   *111*

THE SIX PILLARS   *119*

SHIHŌ-NAGE: *Gratitude*   *120*

IRIMI: *Entering*   *122*

KAITEN: *Open and Turn*   *125*

KOKYŪ: *Breath Power*   *129*

OSAE-WAZA: *Firm Control*   *133*

USHIRO-WAZA: *Sixth Sense*   *137*

RIAI: *The Integrated System*   *139*

APPENDIXES
KOTOTAMA
THE SECRET SOUNDS OF AIKIDŌ   *145*

Suggested Reading   *149*

Credits   *150*

PREFACE

Morihei Ueshiba, the founder of Aikidō, once said to a group of his senior students, "Come to the *dōjō* tomorrow morning at 5:00 AM and I will tell you the secrets of Aikidō." The students arrived the next day at that early hour, eagerly anticipating the revelation of a secret that would render them invincible like the master—then they would be able to throw ten opponents at once and pin even the strongest adversary with a single finger. Morihei sat the students down and then let the secrets of Aikidō well out of him. Employing vibrant symbolism, intriguing allegory, and free-ranging association, Morihei expounded for more than an hour on the creation of the universe, the animating power of the spirit-sounds, the subtle alchemy of fire and water, the necessity of calming one's spirit and returning to the Source, the transforming nature of mind and body purification, and other mysteries. Suddenly he smiled gently and concluded, "Those are the secrets of Aikidō." Morihei bowed deeply to the *dōjō* shrine, turned to bow to his students, and then whisked himself out of the room. All of the students were bewildered by Morihei's words, and those who had longed to be taught some amazing trick or be given the words to a magic formula were resentful: "He didn't show us anything—not a single technique or anything concrete to use!"

What Morihei had done was reveal Aikidō as a deep and wonderful epiphany, not merely a system of throws, locks, and pins. If one fails to grasp the heart of Aikidō, Morihei was telling them, the techniques will never come alive. Like all good masters, Morihei illuminated just one corner of the Truth, leaving it up to the students to plumb the depths of Aikidō on their own.

The Secrets of Aikidō is such an exploration of the different dimensions of Morihei's teaching and how Aikidō relates to other spiritual and cultural traditions. There are not a lot of details in this book—some techniques are shown but always as illustrations of more profound inner principles—because one of the meanings of *Aikidō* is "resonance." It is hoped that the ideas and illustrations presented here will strike certain chords in my readers' hearts, which they will then be able to express in their own ways, based on their own experiences. Aikidō is, ultimately, a grand harmony orchestrated from a melodious blend of unique individual tones.

Since the *The Secrets of Aikidō* presupposes a considerable degree of familiarity with the practice of Aikidō and the life and and teaching of Morihei, the book will be more accessible and useful if the reader employs the other works listed in "Suggested Reading" as stepping-stones.

I am most grateful to Kisshomaru Ueshiba, Morihei's son and present Grandmaster of Aikidō, for permission to reproduce photographs from the Ueshiba family collection and to quote from Morihei's writings. Hidenobu Hozumi, Director of the Banshōkan in Sendai, kindly allowed me to photograph some scenes in his beautiful, traditional Shintō-style *dōjō*. Heartfelt thanks go to Alan Nagahisa, of Ohana Aikidō in Hawaii, who took many action shots of me and to Walther von Krenner, who provided a number of photographs of Morihei from his personal collection. I also wish to thank Toma Rosenzweig, who supplied some shots of Morihei; my *uke* in the photos (Hugh Gribben, Sean Collins, Yosuke Yoshida, Jorge Delva, and Roger Kwok); and those who helped with the photography (Justin Lahart, Paul McLaughlin, and Kyle Fujisue).

PART ONE

STUDY OF THE WAY
THE MYSTERIES OF AIKIDŌ

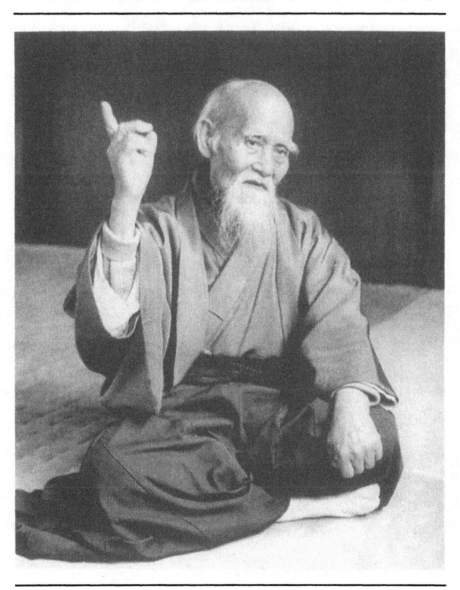

AIKIDŌ
The Way of Harmony

Aiki, THE FIRST HALF OF THE WORD *AIKIDŌ,* CONSISTS OF THE two Chinese characters *ai,* meaning "to come together, to blend, to join, to harmonize," and *ki,* a word with manifold meanings that include (as in this case) "spirit" and "disposition." *Aiki* has always been a central theme of Asian philosophy, but Morihei declared: "My interpretation of *aiki* is much broader than those of the past." Morihei defined *aiki* in the following ways:

> *Aiki* is the universal principle that brings all things together; it is the optimal process of unification and harmonization that operates in all realms, from the vastness of space to the tiniest atoms.

> *Aiki* reflects the grand design of the cosmos; it is the life force, an irresistible power that binds the material and spiritual aspects of creation. *Aiki* is the flow of nature.

> *Aiki* signifies the union of body and spirit and is a manifestation of that truth. Further, *aiki* enables us to harmonize heaven, earth, and humankind as one.

> *Aiki* means "to live together in harmony," in a state of mutual accord. *Aiki* is the ultimate social virtue. It is the power of reconciliation, the power of love.

Morihei's vision of *aiki* corresponds closely to the notions of *integritas* (wholeness) and *consonantia* (harmony) in Western philosophy. Integration—between body and spirit, self and other, humankind and nature, truth and beauty—is a condition that all people should strive for, and integrity is a moral state as well: those who are whole can act in the best and fairest manner.

Consonantia (*harmonia* in Greek) is "a fitting together." The wise ones of the West, too, perceived the harmony of the spheres and the process in which all elements orchestrate themselves into the greater whole. As Hippocrates wrote, "All things are in sympathy." In present-day physics this is stated as: "The amount of positive energy in the universe is exactly equal to the amount of negative energy; the universe is, and always has been, a perfectly balanced energy system."

The intuition that "all things are in sympathy" was a common belief in both East and West. Tragically, modern civilization has been poisoned by the misguided contention of some that life is nothing more than an intense rivalry between species and only the fittest can survive. Life is always a trial, and people need to be physically and mentally fit to get along—this is one of the reasons we practice Aikidō—but the pernicious view that existence is a constant battle against foes that must be totally subjugated or annihilated is a direct cause of much of the exploitation and destruction of both humankind and the environment that has surfaced violently in the nineteenth and twentieth centuries.

The emphasis on being the "victor," whatever the means and whatever the cost, has largely obliterated the noble ideal of "sportsmanship" in contemporary athletics. Morihei wrote: "Sports nowadays are only good for physical exercise—they do not train the whole person. The practice of *aiki,* on the other hand, fosters valor, sincerity, fidelity, goodness, and beauty, as well as making the body strong and healthy." In traditional Aikidō there are no formal contests, and thus no "winners" and no "losers." This position is very difficult for certain people to accept, and even some of Morihei's closest disciples disagreed with the master on this point—they insisted on establishing some sort of competition, either in the form of Judō-style matches or Olympic-style point-system contests.

Morihei, though, maintained to the end that *aiki* is cooperation. In each Aikidō exercise, the partners take turns being the attacker and the defender, the winner and the loser. In this manner, a trainee learns much from experiencing both sides of the Aikidō equation. Onlookers (and sometimes students themselves) often remark, "Aikidō techniques only work if your partner cooperates." That is exactly the point. Rinjirō Shirata Sensei used to explain *aiki* thus: "Living in harmony, let us join hands and reach the finish line together."

Aiki, as a healing agent, connotes resuscitation and revitalization. The best doctors in any culture understand that a proper diagnosis largely depends on being in tune with the patient in order to sense what really ails him or her. Then an appropriate remedy can be suggested. (In the old days in Japan, a type of *aiki* was used to resuscitate people knocked unconscious in accidents or in comas from illnesses.) Morihei often spoke of the health-giving, restorative properties of *aiki* training: "After a good workout, you should have more energy than you began with!"

There is another meaning of *aiki* that is central to true harmony: the consummate union of a man and a woman, a blissful state of complete physical and spiritual intimacy. (In Chinese sex manuals, *aiki* was the term used for the ultimate sexual experience.) The natural and pure integration of male and female principles is at the heart of all creation. Libido should not be mistaken for mere concupiscence but rather should be understood as a sincere yearning for integration and fulfillment. Male and female remain barren until united; the desire to cleave together as one, to restore the primordial unity, is a key goal of Aikidō (and all other arts).

Similarly, there is a kind of *aiki* embryology: the ideal child is conceived when both parents are in total harmony, truly as one in body and soul. If the parents remain in accord during the pregnancy, the fetus is nurtured with *aiki,* a quality that beats in the mother's heart and flows in her blood.

Technically, *aiki* is "perfect timing." In the *dōjō* one attempts to blend smoothly with the attacking force, applying just the right amount of movement, balance, and power. In everyday existence, one tries similarly to fit right in, responding to the various challenges of life with a keen *aiki* sense.

Dō, the second half of the word *Aikidō,* symbolizes both a particular "path" that one treads and a universal "way" of philosophical principles. Those who walk the path of Aikidō wear a special type of outfit, meditate in a certain manner, and practice distinctive forms. This is the cultural *path* of Aikidō, the context of practice based on the ideals and classical techniques of the Founder, Morihei. The *way* of Aikidō involves the broader spectrum of life—how we interact with other human beings outside the narrow world of the *dōjō,* how we relate to society as a whole, and how we deal with nature.

In this sense, Aikidō is Tantra, a knitting together of the macro- and microcosms. The basic truth of Tantra is: "All that exists in the universe exists within one's own body. What is here is there; what is not here is nowhere." In Western gnosticism this is expressed as: "When you make the above like the below, and when you make the male and female as one, you will enter the Kingdom" *(Gospel of Thomas),* or more succinctly: "As above, so below." In Morihei's idiom this is stated as *ware soku uchū,* "I am (we are) the universe!" By cultivating our individual body and soul through Aikidō practice, by acquiring true perception and creating real acts, we learn to live cosmically.

Aikidō is also yoga, a "yoke" that unifies, conjoins, and harnesses us to higher principles. The eight limbs of classical yoga parallel the teachings of Morihei's classical Aikidō:

> *Yama,* "ethics," primary of which is *ahiṃsā,* "nonviolence." In Morihei's words, "Those who seek competition are making a grave mistake. To smash, injure, or destroy is the worst sin a human being can commit."

> *Niyama,* "discipline," in Aikidō is termed *tanren* (forging): "The purpose of training is to tighten up the slack, toughen the body, and polish the spirit."

> *Āsana,* "graceful postures." Sometimes it is helpful for trainees to think of Aikidō movements not as lethal martial art techniques but as *āsana,* physical postures that link the practitioner to higher truths. Like *āsana,* Aikidō techniques are painful and difficult in the beginning, but eventually they become easier, more stable, and agreeable. Indeed it is said in yoga that "the *āsana* is perfect when the effort to attain it disappears" and "one who masters the *āsana* conquers the three worlds." Morihei taught: "Functioning harmoniously together, right and left give birth to all techniques. The four limbs of the body are the four pillars of heaven."

> *Prāṇāyāma,* "breath control," is necessary to partake of the breath of the universe: "Breathe in and let yourself soar to the ends of the universe; breathe out and bring the cosmos back inside. Next, breathe up all the fecundity of earth. Finally, blend the breath of heaven and the breath of earth with your own, becoming the Breath of Life itself."

> *Pratyāhāra* connotes "freedom from bewilderment," a withdrawal from the distraction of the senses, a mind that is steadfast and imperturbable. Regarding this, Morihei instructed: "Do not stare into the eyes of your opponent: he may mesmerize you. Do not fix your gaze on his sword: he may intimidate you. Do not focus on your opponent at all: he may absorb your energy."

> *Dhāraṇā,* "fixing the mind," is also known as *ekāgratā,* "keeping the one point," a well-known concept in Aikidō circles: "If you are centered, you can move freely. The physical center is your belly; if

your mind is set there as well, you are assured of victory in any endeavor."

Dhyāna, "meditation," is a state of penetrating insight and clear vision: "Cast off limiting thoughts and return to true emptiness. Stand in the midst of the Great Void."

Samādhi, "total absorption," goes even further. In *samādhi,* the distinction between knower and known dissolves, a transfiguration that Morihei expressed as "I am the universe!" Morihei's supernatural powers originated in his all-absorbing *aiki samādhi,* and his eccentric behavior likewise was characteristic of the highest levels of yoga—a kind of divine madness that transcended time and space. "If you do not blend with the emptiness of the Pure Void, you will not find the path of *aiki.*"

Morihei's teaching was summed up in the phrase *Takemusu Aiki. Take* stands for "valor and bravery"; it represents the irrepressible and indomitable courage to live. *Musu* typifies birth, growth, accomplishment, fulfillment. It is the creative force of the cosmos, responsible for the production of all that nourishes life. *Takemusu Aiki* is code for "the boldest and most creative existence!"

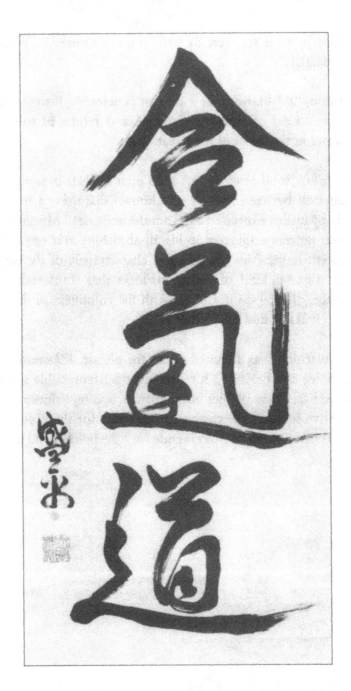

AI-KI-DŌ, "The Way of Harmony," brushed by Morihei in his eighties. The calligraphy itself is a manifestation of *aiki:* balanced, stable, and vibrant.

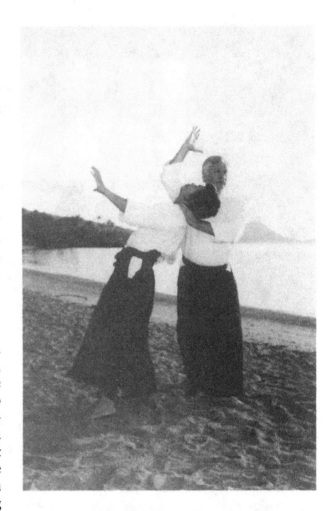

Aiki signifies harmony and integration—between body and soul, self and other, humankind and nature. When practiced properly in a good environment, *aiki* is an inexhaustible source of energy and love.

Zen painting by Kaizan (c. early 20th century) of a chrysanthemum and an orchid with the inscription, "Gentlemen do not fight." The chrysanthemum and the orchid are two of the "Four Gentlemen" (the other two are the plum blossom and the bamboo). That well-mannered people refrain from unseemly arguments is a Confucian sentiment; Zen and Aikidō further imply that gentlemen and gentlewomen do not compete or become jealous—each individual is splendid in his or her own right. Morihei always encouraged his students to bring forth the fragrant flower of their unique inner beauty.

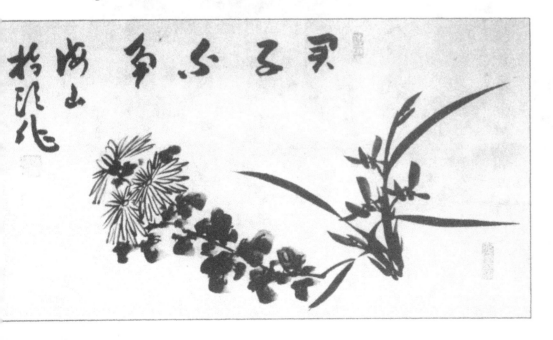

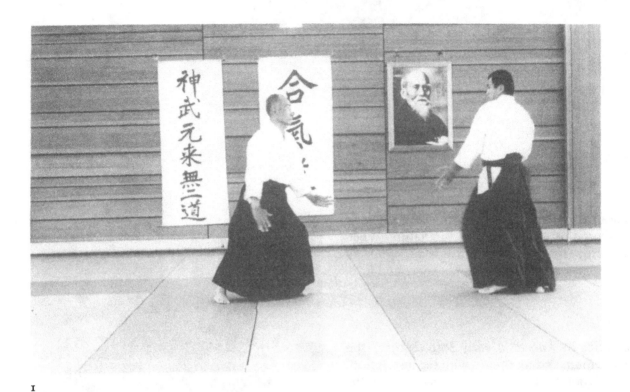

1

Rinjirō Shirata Sensei demonstrating *aiki* timing: as the attack is developing, he responds with a flexible *aiki* stance (1); rather than colliding with the oncoming force, he glides smoothly past it, directing it up and then down (2, 3); even though the actual movement is completed, Shirata Sensei remains subtly linked to his partner (4).

3

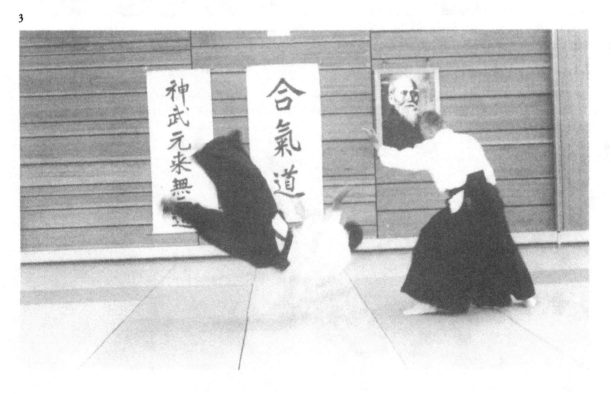

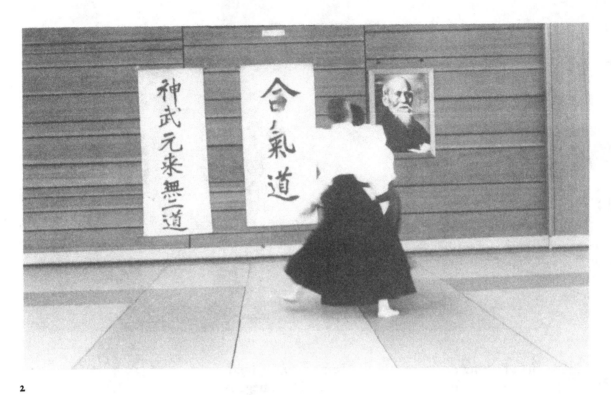

2

4

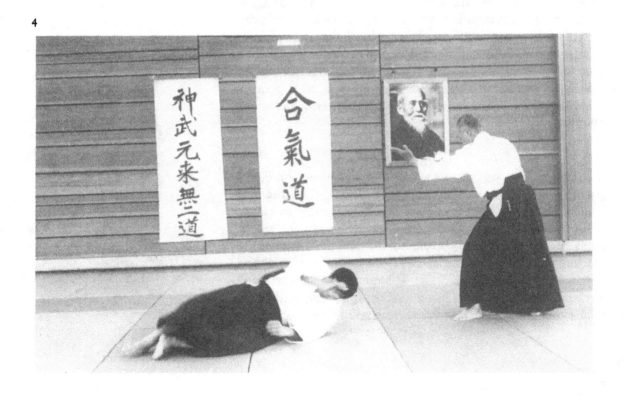

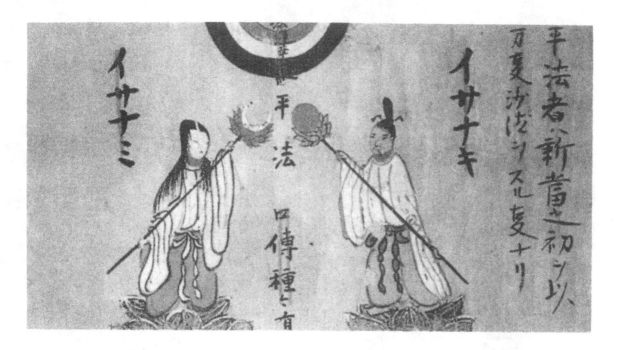

Izanami (*left,* holding up the moon) and Izanagi (*right,* holding up the sun), two Shintō gods of creation. This image is from a secret transmission scroll of the Shinkage school of swordsmanship. In Aikidō as well, the harmonious functioning of Izanami (mother) and Izanagi (father), sexually and spiritually, symbolizes the cooperative nature of the universe. Morihei often utilized the symbols of Izanami and Izanagi in his teaching: "Izanami is the female, receptive element associated with water, centrifugal force, and the right side of things; Izanagi is the male, active element associated with fire, centripetal force, and the left side of things." Morihei hoped that each woman would realize her potential as a goddess of compassion and each man his potential as a victorious buddha.

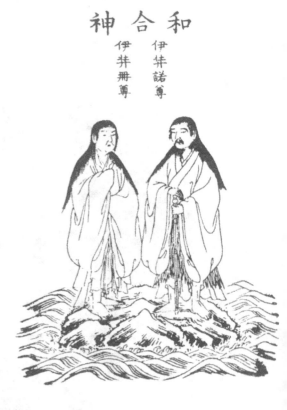

Izanami and Izanagi are also known as *wagō no kami,* the gods of harmony, again representing the ideal of true and fruitful intimacy. The two deities are standing on the island of Onogoro, the name of which may be interpreted as "within one's heart." Some *budō* scrolls stated that the secret of the martial arts was to become as close to your opponent as "two lovers in sexual embrace." The Western equivalent of *wagō no kami* would be the Greek deities Aphrodite and Ares, whose daughter Harmonia weaved the veil of the universe.

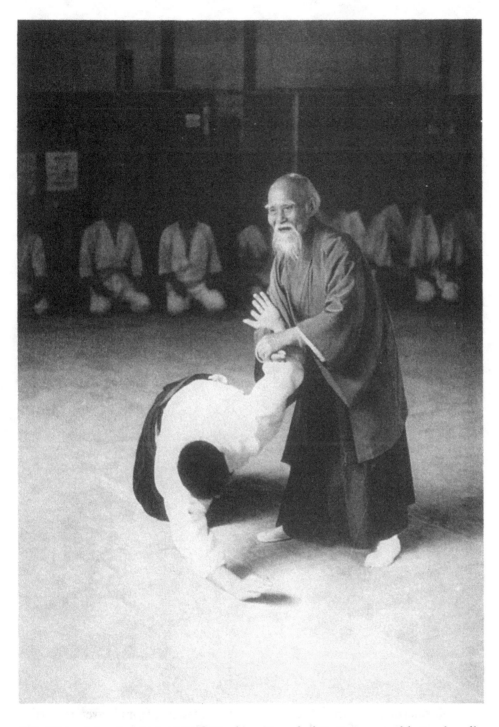

Morihei maintained that "*aiki* is love," and that it is possible to handle aggression with a smile. The supreme challenge of a warrior is to turn an enemy's fearful wrath into harmless laughter.

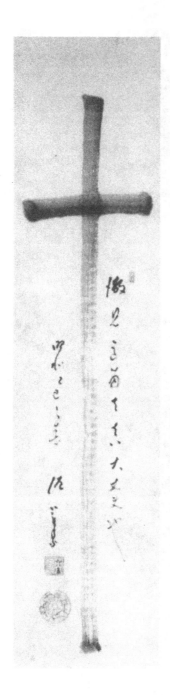

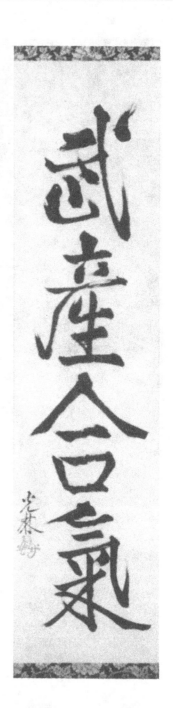

Left: Morihei characterized Aikidō as "a cross reaching from heaven to earth, linking *yin* and *yang,* fire and water." The inscription on this painting by the Zen Master Mamiya Eshū (1871–1945) says, "Once you grasp this, everything will be all right!"

Right: Takemusu Aiki, brushed by Shirata Sensei.

KOTOTAMA

THE LANGUAGE OF THE GODS

KOTOTAMA, "WORD-SPIRIT," IS A JAPANESE TERM, BUT THE existence of a pristine language voiced directly by the gods of creation is a notion deeply imbedded in global culture. The *fiat lux*—"Let there be light!"—of Genesis (1:3) is a *kototama,* in which pronouncement and deed are simultaneous. The name Adam, too, is a *kototama: A* = ascent, the east; *D* = descent, the west; *A* = arctic, the north; and *M* = meridian, the south. That is, as the first man, Adam's word-spirit embraced all four directions of the universe. God taught Adam the true language—each sound corresponded exactly to each object—and he was thus able to name all the plants and animals of the world. (In medieval England it was believed that boy babies at birth uttered the cry "Ah, Ah" for "Adam," but girl babies cried "Ee, Ee" for "Eve.") The old-time prophets of Israel were well aware of the tremendous potency of *kototama:* the mighty war cry of Joshua and his army shattered the walls of Jericho (Joshua 6:20). Some Jewish Kabbalists believe that the text of the Torah is deliberately garbled; if intoned precisely, the *kototama* of the Torah is so powerful that it would enable a human being to create worlds, raise the dead, and perform other miracles.

The Sufis of Islam composed mystic texts consisting entirely of Arabic-style *kototama*—the Abjad scheme, a hidden tongue of mathematical precision and esoteric meaning. Also in Islam, there is the practice of reciting the "Ninety-Nine Names of Allah." One such name, for example, is Al-Fattaḥ, "The Opener," a *kototama* that "opens one's heart and eliminates all obstacles." African tribes such as the Dogon firmly believe that speech itself was the original act of creation, and they consider farming, weaving, and making love to be expressions of that speech.

The most prominent example of the *kototama* principle in the West occurs at the beginning of the Gospel of Saint John: "In the beginning was the Word." *Logos* (*verbum* in Latin) is rich with meaning: "order," "pattern," "blueprint," "ratio," "*oratio*" (discourse and articulation), "reason," "principal cause," and "harmony between opposites." *Logos* can also be interpreted as "perfect consonance," the simultaneous and harmonious blending of sounds. In this case, the harmony of *aiki* is actualized as the sounds of speech and music.

The sounds of speech and music have a healing dimension, another extension of *aiki* principles. The Greek philosopher and mathematician Pythagoras promoted the study of the "music of the spheres" in his academy, beginning and ending the lessons with songs, which he believed could cure the mental and physical ailments of his pupils. In English, too, we have the ideal of "a sound mind in a sound body," which is to say that "being in tune leads to wholeness and strength." It is well known that plants clearly respond to musical *kototama*—they flourish when exposed to Indian ragas and European classical music but are likely to wither and die if given a heavy dose of hard rock.

In Hindu thought this principle was stated as "Whatever the gods do, they do by song." (Native Americans believed the same thing: "The Great Spirit gave humankind songs and drum beats to keep in touch with the Divine Presence.") Sound—embodied by the sacred symbol OM—shapes and holds matter together; everything has a voice. Creation proceeds from the subtle to the gross through sound (*nāda*); variations in the concentration and wavelength of the nuclear seed-sounds give birth to what human beings perceive as light, volume, and structure. (Or, as a quantum physicist would say, "All matter is vibration.") In Buddhist sūtras—which begin with the declaration, "Thus I have heard"—the state of nirvāṇa was sometimes defined as the harmonious blending of all primordial sounds: "When Buddha appeared in a place, all animals trumpeted, neighed, and mooed with delight; all birds chirped happily in unison; all ornaments clinked together melodiously; and all musical instruments sounded as one."

In old Tibet, work equaled song. The Tibetans had a distinct song for every kind of occupation—plowing, sowing, harvesting, grinding grain, loading for market, calculating the bill, rock-breaking, roadwork, house-building, sewing, weaving, on and on. Without the animating presence of songs, little could be accomplished.

Morihei formulated his understanding of *kototama* within the context of his own culture. He learned deeply the science of sound taught in Shingon Buddhism and Ōmoto-kyō. Onisaburō Deguchi, the cofounder of Ōmoto-kyō, told Morihei: "Every human being is a living shrine, a miniature universe. If you desire to know the truth of heaven and earth, and discern the grand design of creation, study the gods you have within. If you train sincerely with a pure heart, you can actually hear the sounds that sustain creation."

After many years of intense study, Morihei presented his vision of *kototama* to his disciples. The "Big Bang" in Morihei's scheme is the nuclear syllable SU. This is the point of creation, the center of all existence. Usually in Asian thought A is considered the seed-syllable supreme, but in certain systems such as Morihei's, SU is held to be a more likely candidate because it represents the actual act of breathing, not merely the act of opening the mouth, as with A. (Even in English, *S* is pronounced with a more forceful expenditure of breath than *A*.) Morihei explained the evolution of the cosmos in this manner:

> There was no heaven, no earth, no universe, just empty space. In this vast emptiness, a single point suddenly manifest itself. From that point steam, smoke, and mist spiraled forth in a luminous sphere and the *kototama* SU was born. As SU expanded circularly up and down, left and right, nature and breath began, clear and uncontaminated. Breath developed into life and sound appeared. SU is the "Word" mentioned in the Christian Bible.

In Shintō mythology SU is identified with Ame-no-minaka-nushi-no-kami, "Lord Deity of Heaven's Center." From this single point of creation evolved two primordial generative forces called in Shintō *takami-musubi-no-kami* and *kami-no-musubi-no-kami*. In other systems these two pivots of creation are designated by such terms as Śiva-Śākti; *yang-yin;* fire-water; Sky Father–Earth Mother; centripetal force–centrifugal force.

On the microcosmic level, Morihei placed SU in the midpoint of our being. In the womb, human life begins with a single sphere that, through the interaction of the two generative forces, passes through every form of organic structure, ranging from the lowest (amoeba) to the highest (a man or a woman). This means that a human being actually experiences the sum total of sentient existence in the womb—a fact that most people have forgotten by the time they are grown.

As SU continued to expand, the *kototama* U appeared. Simultaneously U spun into the *kototama* YU and MU and extended out into the *kototama* A-O-U-E-I. The syllable YU means "there is," "something," "yes"; MU signifies "is not," "nothing," "no." Combined, they are pronounced UMU, the Japanese word for "birth." This indicates the fact that for life to appear, there must be an integration of the physical and the spiritual; existence is a balance of form (the body) and emptiness (the soul). A-O-U-E-I are the *kototama* that vivify the world. The symbolism of each *kototama* may be briefly stated as follows:

> A extends up. It stands for actualization from *atama* (head) to *ashi* (foot). A is the first among sounds, the mother of all letters, and it is centered around the mouth and throat.

> O moves down, and the tension between it and A creates physical forms. O is thus identified with the outside of things, the "shell." O is centered near the heart.

> U returns to itself, giving birth, moving things, making it possible for people to obtain life. (Intriguingly, the vowel *U* in English also has connotations of "elemental deepness," "source of being," and "procreative secret.") U originates deep in the belly.

> E branches out to become the channels, wrapping, and limbs of life forms. E is felt spreading throughout the body.

> I is the life force, full-spirited breath. I vibrates powerfully, and it is projected out from the body.

From these five vowels sprang the rest of the Japanese alphabet, all together seventy-five sounds (arranged in the ancient order):

A	KA	SA	TA	NA	HA	MA	YA	RA	WA
O	KO	SO	TO	NO	HO	MO	YO	RO	(W)O
U	KU	SU	TSU	NU	FU	MU	YU	RU	(W)U
E	KE	SE	TE	NE	HE	ME	(Y)E	RE	(W)E
I	KI	SHI	CHI	NI	HI	MI	(Y)I	RI	(W)I
			GA	ZA	DA		BA	PA	
			GO	ZO	DO		BO	PO	
			GU	ZU	(T)ZU		BU	PU	
			GE	ZE	DE		BE	PE	
			GI	JI	(C)JI		BI	PI	

These sounds are molded into *kotoba*, words containing real meaning, and *kotomuke*, soothing speech that brings peace.

How did Morihei actually put into practice the science of *kototama*? Morihei used to seclude himself for much of the morning, losing himself in the experience of the *kototama* SU and listening to the vibration of A-O-U-E-I.

Prior to actual training, Morihei typically employed the *kototama* o to prepare himself. Pronounced with full concentration of body and spirit, the
sound o is a resonance of the universal grand design; Morihei felt that o and
the other *kototama* activated the hidden powers of the universe and put even
deities under one's control. (The *kototama* o is often pronounced in other
Shintō rites to summon the gods, and Japanese fishing folk and woman divers
chant O-O-O-O to calm stormy seas.)

Since Morihei was able to display incredible powers, it may be assumed
that he really did strike the right chord with his *kototama*. But how are students to make use of this vital element of Aikidō culture? Although Morihei
talked constantly about *kototama*, it was a private practice for him ("I'm the
only one in Japan still doing real *kototama*," he used to say), and he gave no
real instructions. *Kototama* was something that each person had to explore
for him- or herself.* Any language can be used, since every human tongue
possesses effective word-spirits.

There will be some people who disagree with this last statement (including
Morihei, who inherited the culturally conditioned Ōmoto-kyō conceit that
the sound su occurs only in the Japanese language). This kind of linguistic
provincialism—"Our tongue is the best and most beautiful, beyond compare
with any other"—was (and is) still common, but as we learn more about the
universal dimensions of word-spirit, it will be impossible to seriously maintain such shortsighted views. When confronted with the arguments of linguistic purists, I like to relate this enlightening tale from Tibet:

A pious but uneducated old peasant woman devoted herself to nursing the
sick. Her prayers, badly pronounced and grammatically incorrect, nonethe-
less had a soothing effect on all those who were ill and under her care. Many
people said that her prayers even effected complete cures of their ailments.
One day her son, who had spent many years in a distant monastery and had
become a formidable scholar, visited the old woman. The son was appalled
at his mother's faulty diction and garbled syntax, so he taught her the proper
sentence structure and standard pronunciation of the prayers. After her son
had gone back to his monastery, the old woman resumed her charitable work.
As she self-consciously stumbled over the right pronunciation of the words,
though, she found that the healing properties of her prayers had vanished.
Once she returned to her old inelegant but heartfelt chants, however, her
miraculous healing powers returned.

A *kototama* is not a magic abracadabra—it is only effective when accompanied by a sincere attitude, genuine compassion, and deep wisdom.

Another important aspect of *kototama* is *kiai*, the battle cry of Aikidō. On
the physical plane, *kiai* is a rousing shout emanating from the belly, reflecting

*See the first appendix for a description of a variety of *kototama* chants.

the harmonization of body and mind; on the spiritual level, *kiai* is the motivating force that shapes firm resolve and full concentration. Morihei's external *kiai*, not surprisingly, was awesome—his shouts could be heard a mile away—while his internal *kiai* enabled him to disarm an attack before it began. Even on his deathbed Morihei's *kiai* was incredibly powerful. Although Morihei was so weak from his final illness that he had to be carried up the stairs, as soon as he entered the shrine room and into a divine presence he stood bolt straight and extended his arms, sending his attendant disciples flying.

Kiai is essential to all the Japanese arts. The tea master Rikyū was said to overflow with *kiai* when he performed a ceremony, and even the most skilled samurai felt that the Rikyū presented no openings for attack. Connoisseurs of sushi insist that they can discern how the raw fish and rice will taste from the quality of *kiai* in the "Welcome!" shouted out by the chef when customers enter his shop. *Kiai*, in short, is the *kototama* of life's energy.

The implementation of *kototama* on a technical level is called *yamabiko*, "mountain echo." Morihei frequently presented his teaching in the form of *waka* poetry, another kind of *kototama* (a parallel found in the Latin *cantare*, meaning both "song" and "incantation"). Regarding *yamabiko*, Morihei sang:

> *Link yourself to*
> *Heaven and earth;*
> *Stand in the very center*
> *With your heart receptive to*
> *The flow of the mountain echo.*

Just as a mountain echo embraces any sound, in any language, in whatever manner it is projected, Aikidō techniques, executed on the highest level, enable one to respond to, embrace, and turn back any challenge regardless of the circumstances.

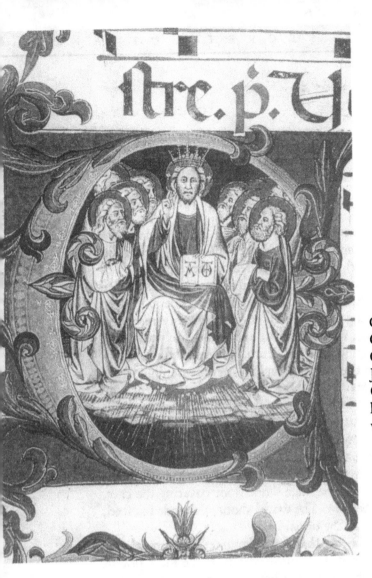

Christ the King bearing the *kototama* Alpha and Omega in his Book of Life. Alpha-Omega is the Christian equivalent of the Sanskrit OM and the Japanese A-UN. In Japanese *kototama* theory, Christ is pronounced *Ki-ri-su-to*, "the One who has completely cut off all ties" to the profane world.

Vibrating Sanskrit sacred syllables represented in the form of a cosmic serpent. The dynamic power of such *kototama* sustains creation and animates all forms of life.

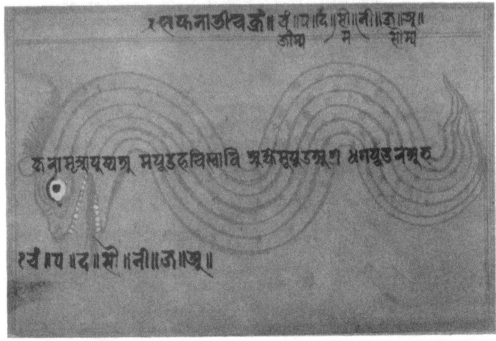

Opposite: Amaterasu emerging from the cave and once again bathing the cosmos in light. Morihei often mentioned the symbolism of this important Shintō mythological tale (*Kojiki* 17). Terribly offended by the impetuous and rude behavior of her brother Susano-o, Amaterasu, the Sun Goddess, sealed herself in a cave, thereby casting heaven into impenetrable darkness. In deep consternation, the rest of the gods gathered in an attempt to lure Amaterasu back to the world. Ame-no-Uzume, who was as voluptuous as she was strong and fierce, began dancing and singing on a big drum. When she started stripping off her clothes (not shown in this demure depiction), the assembled gods burst into mirthful laughter. Amaterasu, who had heretofore spurned all prayers for her return, exclaimed, "I have never heard such wonderful sounds as those." As Amaterasu peeked out from the cave, Ame-no-Uzume (falsely) informed her that the cause of the gay outburst was the discovery of a goddess more brilliant than Amaterasu. Ame-no-Uzume cleverly held up a mirror before Amaterasu, and as the surprised Sun Goddess leaned farther out of the cave, Ame-no-Tajikara-o pulled back the huge stone door covering the cave, grabbed Amaterasu, and pulled her out. The world shone, the gods rejoiced, and Amaterasu agreed to stay out in the open.

Shintō scholars make much of the fact that it was laughter that lured Amaterasu out of hiding—"Laughter, not dark incantations, is the most potent of all *kototama*," a sentiment with which Morihei certainly agreed. Morihei considered himself to be an incarnation of Ame-no-Tajikara-o, the Shintō Hercules and patron saint of sumō wrestlers and other strong men. Morihei often characterized the establishment of Aikidō as "a second opening of the stone door." Prior to training, Morihei would frequently do a *kagura* dance with a *jō*, or fan, in emulation of Ame-no-Uzume's rousing performance that dispelled the world's darkness.

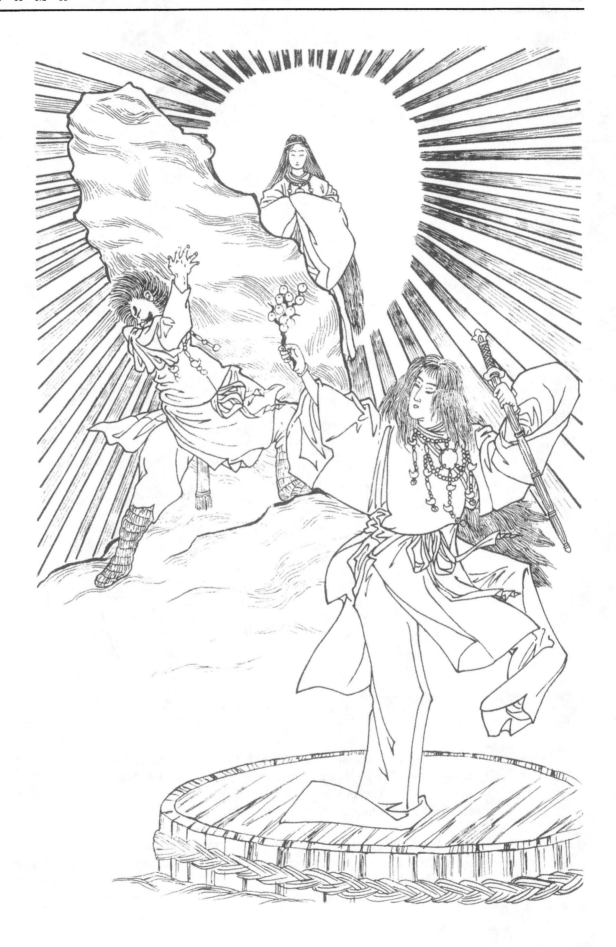

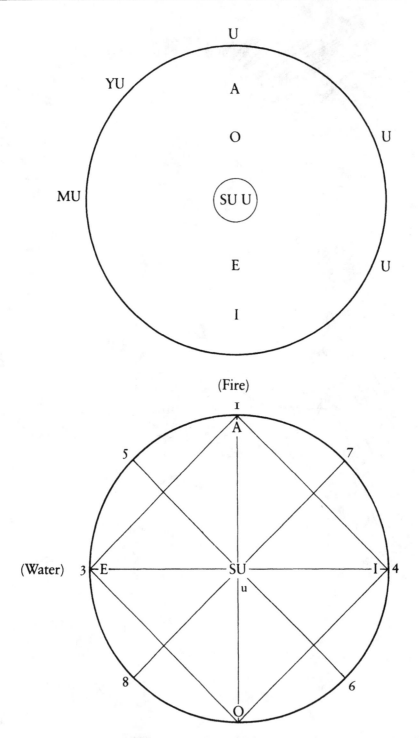

Top: Schematic representation of *kototama* creation. The seed-syllable su u simultaneously spirals forth into U-U-U-YU-MU and A-O-U-E-I. The point in the center represents the Fire-Father-Yang principle, while the outer circle stands for the Water-Mother-Yin principle.

Bottom: A variation of the *kototama* scheme: A–O and E–I extend out from the center, thus creating a tension that brings the world into being. That extension also gives birth to the eight *aiki* powers: movement-stillness, release-solidification, retraction-extension, unification-division.

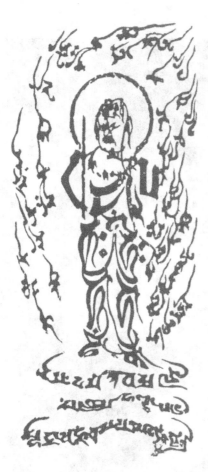

The figure of the protector god Fudō Myō-ō formed by Sanskrit seed-syllables. This is a stunning visual representation of the basic premise of *kototama* belief: our very being vibrates with sacred tones, and all matter is brought into existence through the vehicle of sound.

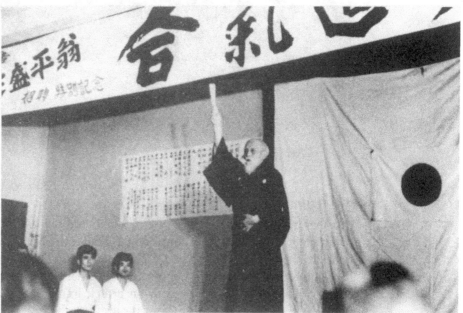

Morihei projecting forth the *kototama* o prior to training. In this case, Morihei spirals his fan up and down, right and left, as he sounds the *kototama* in an elongated note. He places his left hand at the midpoint of his body, the spot where the cosmic seed-syllable su is centered in human beings. This practice, Morihei said, "fires the blood and creates light, heat, and energy."

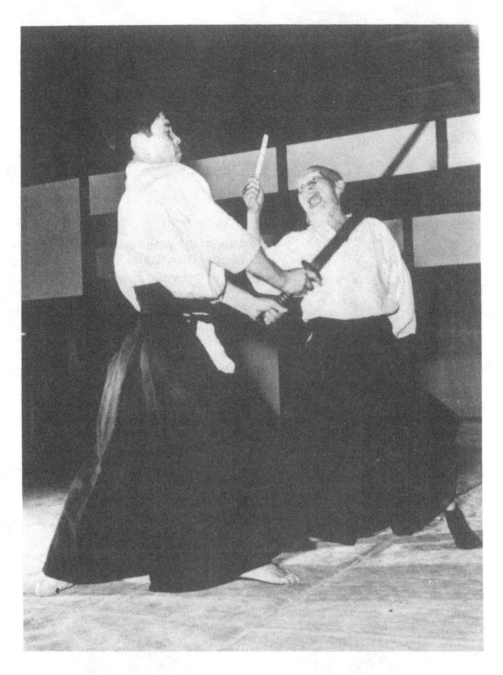

Morihei in the act of emitting one of his incredible *kiai*. His forceful shouts completely unbalanced his opponents (and on occasion extinguished the lights in the *dōjō*). Sometimes Morihei's *kiai* was like a fearful banshee yell, other times like the roar of a hurricane. Morihei also illustrates here the principle of *yamabiko*, responding to an attack immediately and resoundingly, just like a mountain echo.

KAMI
THE DIVINE ALCHEMY OF FIRE AND WATER

ORIHEI TAUGHT THAT AIKIDŌ WAS A FUNCTION OF *KAMI*, the divine alchemy of fire (*ka*) and water (*mi*). (The combination of these two characters can also be read *himitsu*, "holding the key to all secrets.") Fire and water are the two prime elements of outer and inner alchemy, in the East and in the West, and are associated with the polarities of heaven and earth, the sun and the moon, *yang* and *yin*, *logos* and *eros*, hidden and manifest, positive and negative, heart and womb, man and woman. In the Kabbalah, the integration of fire △ and water ▽ is displayed as the Seal of Solomon ✡. In Christianity, humankind is said to be spiritually reborn out of water and fire: "I baptize you with water, but one is coming who will baptize you with the fire of the Holy Spirit" (Luke 3:16).

Like the Jews and Christians, Morihei belived that each human being is a child of god: "If you have the spark of life within, you have divinity." Each person is a *wake-mitama*, an individual part of the great whole, a notion similar to the Hindu concept of *jīva* (personal soul) and *ātman* (universal soul). *Haṭha* is derived from *ha* (sun) and *ṭha* (moon), so *haṭha yoga* is a system that links fire and water, the same goal as Aikidō.

Like the Taoists and Shintoists, Morihei belived that the human soul (*tama*) has two parts. The *kon* element is the "higher soul," the heavenly spirit that endures for eternity; the *haku* element is the "lower soul," the earthly spirit that passes away with the body. The *kon* element represents our higher nature, that which is godlike; the *haku* element is the source of our baser passions and animal drives.

Morihei believed that the *budō* heretofore had been fashioned primarily by the *haku* element. Aikidō, on the other hand, draws its inspiration from the *kon* element, and is one of the harbingers of the coming world civilization. Morihei understood that the way to disarm an attacker is to control the opponent's *haku* with your *kon:* "Defeat your adversaries spiritually by making them realize the folly of their actions."

Following classical Shintō belief, Morihei taught that each individual *tama* has four different aspects: (1) the *kushi-mitama* is the sensitive aspect of the soul, the source of intelligence and wisdom; (2) the *ara-mitama* is the rough aspect of the soul, a source of courage and fortitude if properly channeled, but potentially wild and dangerous if left unchecked; (3) the *nigi-mitama* is the gentle aspect of the soul, the source of empathy and peace; (4) the *sachi-mitama* is the happy aspect of the soul, the source of joy and good tidings. Aikidō training helps develop and refine each of these aspects.

Morihei frequently spoke of the genesis of *kami* in terms of the "red and white jewels" (*akatama-shiratama*). Physiologically, the jewels are the red ova of the female and the white sperm of the male. In Tantra, these are described as *sveta,* the white *bindu* (essence), and *rakta,* the red *bindu.* The conjunction of the red and white jewels creates life, the red jewel evolving into the internal organs, the flesh and the skin, while the white jewel shapes the bones and marrow. The blood must maintain the proper balance of red and white cells to remain healthy. It is interesting to note that in the Tibetan *bardo* teachings, at the time of death the white and red *bindu* distinctly appear (the white emerging in the vicinity of the forehead and the red in the *tanden*), and advanced meditators actually perceive them merging at the heart *chakra.*

The merging of the red and white jewels creates a third *tama,* the clear jewel of pure consciousness (*masumi-tama*). In the alchemical tradition, this state of being is symbolized by the red-and-white rose, the "golden flower" of truth. The proper admixture of the red and white jewels further gives rise to a natural and spontaneous bliss, a truly precious gem.

Kami are also actualized as "gods and goddesses." Shintō has a very broad definition of the divine, and anything that inspires reverence, mystery, or awe is a *kami.* Morihei certainly believed in the existence of all the myriad *kami* found the world over, and they would clearly appear to him. During his morning prayers, Morihei would begin by first paying homage to the sun, and then work his way down through creation, expressing his gratitude to all the *kami* of the animal, vegetable, and mineral worlds. This is not unlike William Blake's contention, "If the doors of perception were cleansed, everything would appear to man as it really is, infinite."

Aikidō is meant to be a bridge between the three realms of manifest, hidden, and divine. The manifest realm is what we can see, hold, taste, smell, and hear; the hidden realm contains time, space, and energy; and the divine lies at the heart of existence, the holy act of creation. In Aikidō training, we must start with the manifest, learning the proper structure of the techniques. After some experience with the manifest forms, one begins to sense the hidden factors of *ki* and *kokyū* power. The last stage is to penetrate even deeper into the first two realms and discover that the techniques are really sacraments, "outer signs of an inner spiritual grace."

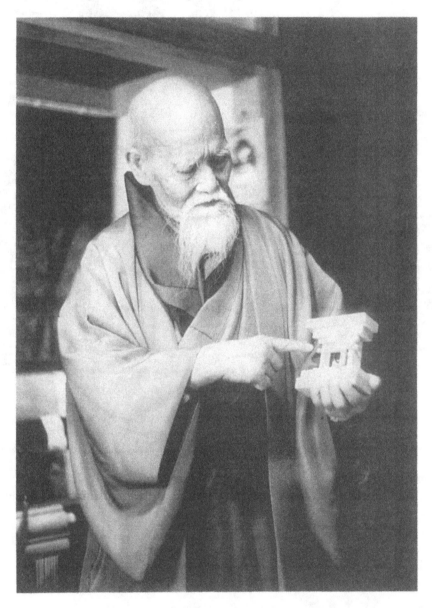

Morihei loved talking about *kami,* large and small. He could sense the Divine all around him and also felt the void of empty ritual. Once on a trip he visited a lavish, newly established shrine. Morihei told his attendant to prepare an offering, but after he bowed to the shrine and prayed for a few minutes, he said to his disciple, "Keep the money. There is no one home here." (The shrine had in fact been erected to attract sightseers, not sincere seekers.)

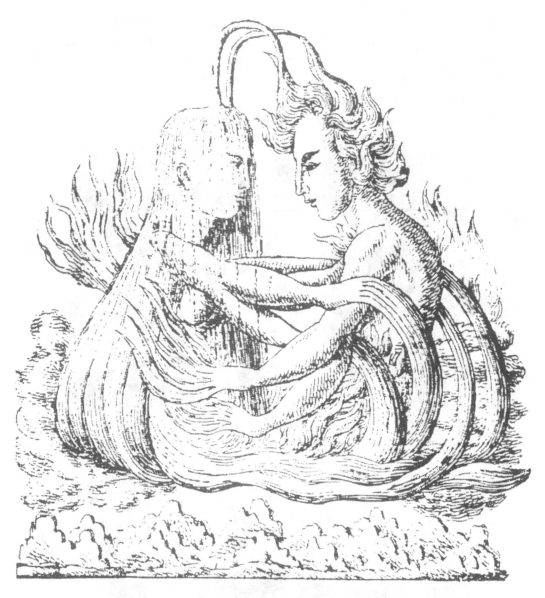

The marriage of fire and water, a common theme of alchemy, East and West. All existence originates and is sustained by the harmonious union of fire and water, male and female.

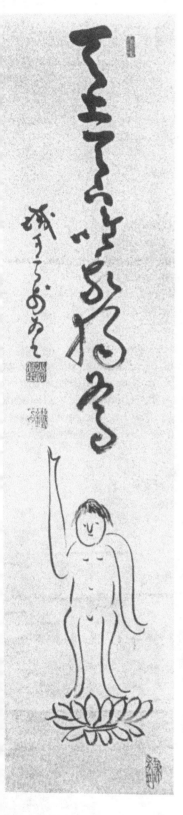

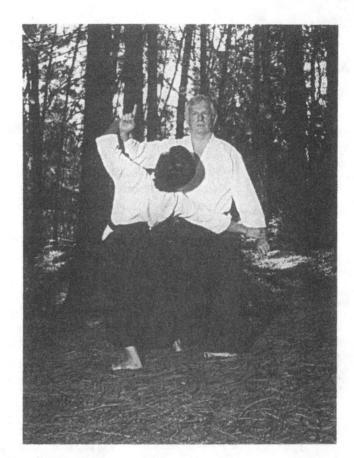

Buddha's stance in Aikidō translates as *tenchi-nage*.

In some places, *kami* is called "buddha-nature." At birth, Gotama Buddha declared himself to be "The Only Honored One in Heaven and Earth." That exclamation is a *kototama* uttered by each newborn human being, and Buddhist enlightenment is the realization of the truth of one's cosmic worth.

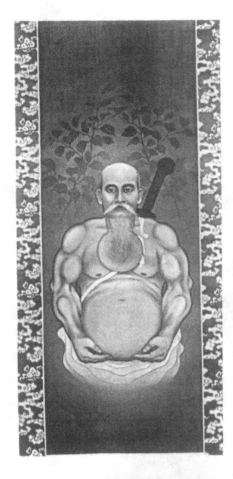

Morihei in transfigured form as a Shintō *kami*. The sword represents bravery and resolution; the mirror symbolizes knowledge and honesty, and his jewel of a belly stands for benevolence and compassion. Every human being has the potential to realize true and unique divinity, and Morihei intended Aikidō to be a vehicle for just that purpose.

The Aiki Shrine Morihei had built in Iwama. The Divine is everywhere but it helps to have something tangible to remind us of our true purpose in life. Morihei dedicated the Aiki Shrine to his forty-three favorite deities—the same number of triangles in the *Sri Yantra*, the most powerful image in Hindu Tantra. Every *dōjō* should be a shrine, "a place where earth is transmuted into gold."

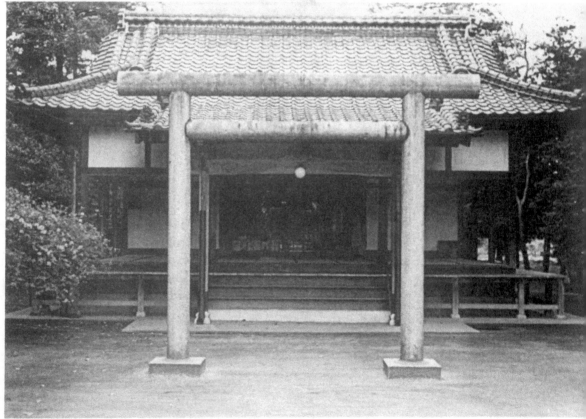

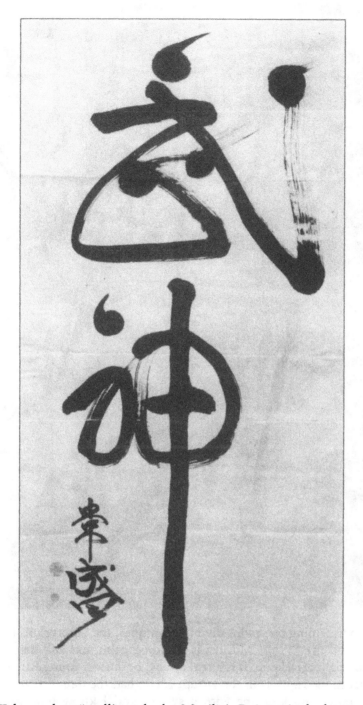

Bushin (Take-no-kami) calligraphy by Morihei. *Bujutsu* is the lowest level of technical fighting; *budō* is the middle level of refinement; and *bushin* is the highest level of spiritual communion.

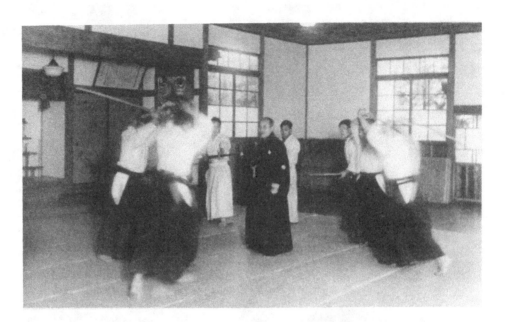

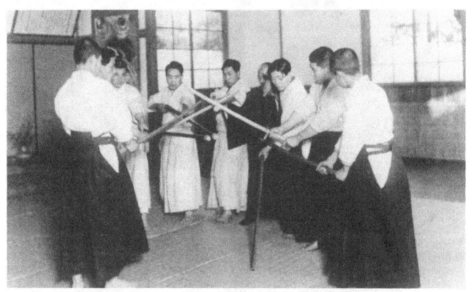

Morihei performing one of his divine techniques, the "marvelous functioning of water and fire." *Top:* Morihei is standing calm and still despite the onslaught of eight attackers. (It is a real attack, because a young Rinjirō Shirata, second from the right, is in the group; I have had the daunting experience of Shirata Sensei attacking me with a sword, and I know how strongly and swiftly he could strike.) *Bottom:* In a flash, Morihei somehow safely removes himself from the circle of attackers—this is a real *ninja* technique, and it is done not through stealth but through the power of enlightened experience.

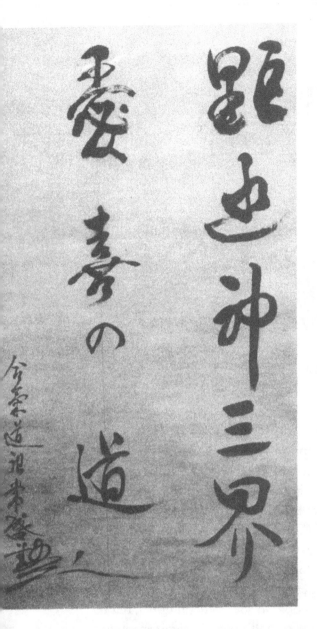
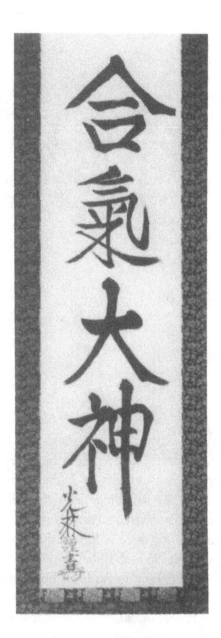

Left: "The Three Realms of Manifest, Hidden, and Divine: Loving and Joyous Path of Aiki," brushed by Morihei. Sporting freely in the three realms leads to a natural joy and affection. In India, there are orders of Rāmānandī ascetics whose yoga practice consists of sacred wrestling. Among these yogis, the mark of a true wrestler is one "who is always happy and takes pleasure in existence."

Right: Aiki Ō-Kami, the "Great Spirit of Aiki," brushed by Rinjirō Shirata. Morihei has returned to the Source, but his *tama* remains with us as Aiki Ō-Kami.

KI
UNIVERSAL ENERGY

CRUCIAL TO THE MAKEUP OF ASIAN CULTURES, *KI* (*CH'I* IN CHInese) has become a familiar concept in the West as well recently. *Ki,* however, is not easy to define in any language. *Ki* is the active agent of creation: "Myriad things bear the *yin* and embrace the *yang,* and through *ki* achieve harmony." Thus, *ki* is synonymous with the very life force itself: "If there is *ki,* there is life. If there is no *ki,* there is death." As an animating principle, *ki* makes the world function: it sustains the wind and rain, it can be felt as heat and cold, it flows in the blood, and it even shapes mountains and rivers. In this sense, *ki* is universal energy.

Morihei discussed the cosmic principles of *ki* in such general terms, but he also used the word to describe more specific conditions. *Ki* signifies vitality and health as expressed in the Japanese word *genki,* "original *ki.*" The practice of Aikidō, Morihei taught his disciples, fosters this original *ki* and keeps one well and vital. One should also learn how to focus *ki:* "Strength resides where one's *ki* is concentrated and stable; confusion and maliciousness reign when *ki* stagnates." As mentioned in chapter 1, *ki* also indicates one's "disposition" toward things. A positive *ki* attitude is essential for mental and physical health. Still another meaning of *ki* is "sensitivity," with perception of forces that cannot be seen with the eyes—such things as electric current and sound waves on the physical plane, and auras on the spiritual plane.

Ki is a prime factor in all the martial arts of Asia. In China, cultivation of *ch'i* is the basis of every school and style; in Japanese *budō, aiki* ("blending of *ki*") and *kiai* ("projection of *ki*") were everything, as we can see in this tale from the nineteenth century:

A young swordsman named Shirai went to challenge the old master Terada. Other swordsmen swore that sparks flew from the end of Terada's wooden sword, and Shirai, upon facing Terada, found that this was no rumor—he was jolted by a shock of *ki* power and was frozen to the spot. Shirai became Takeda's faithful disciple and eventually fathomed the mysteries of *ki*. When opponents come forward Shirai assumed a *ki*-filled stance and stymied them with a surge of *ki* pouring forth from the tip of his *bokken*. He was unbeatable.

In more modern times, Morihei displayed similar miraculous powers even when he was old and seemingly frail. Once in the *dōjō*, Morihei would summon up, concentrate, and project his *ki* so forcefully that his *uke* would be sent flying.

While it is possible to perform certain exercises to foster *ki,* and to "test" for it, Morihei recommended letting *ki* power develop naturally and fully within the context of regular Aikidō training.

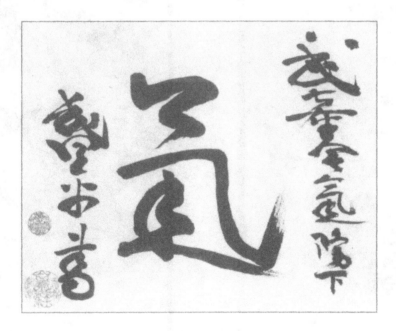

Ki, brushed by Morihei. Along the right-hand side Morihei has written *Takemusu Aiki Koka* (*Morihei sho,* "written by Morihei," is to the left), so the meaning of the calligraphy is "*Takemusu Aiki* has descended and its energy can be felt everywhere." The calligraphy also exhibits a wonderful vital beauty that emanates from the flow of *ki* in the brushstrokes. William Blake wrote, "Energy is eternal delight," and we can sense Morihei's *aiki* elation in this piece. Any great work of art derives much of its beauty from the presence of *ki*.

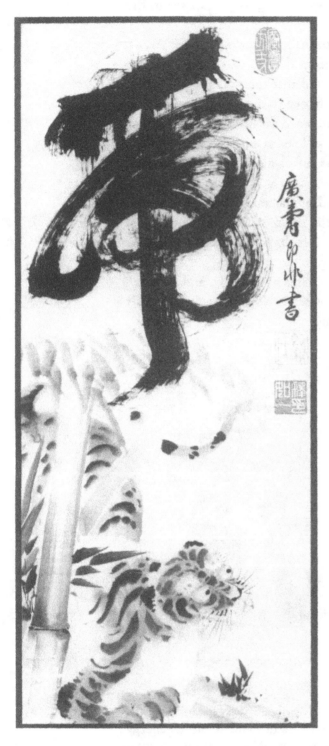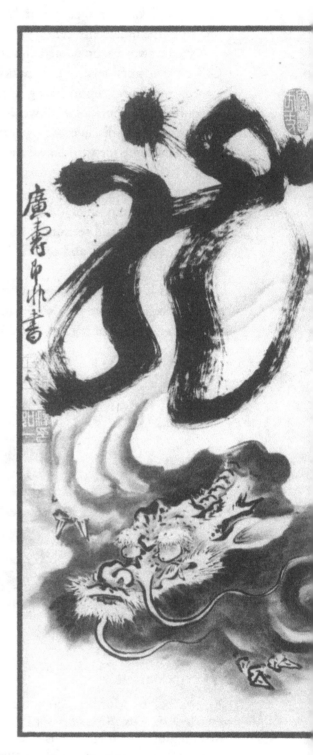

Zen painting in two scrolls by Ōbaku Sokuhi (1616–1671), depicting *ki* power in the world of nature. The *yang* tiger of earth faces off against the *yin* dragon of heaven, generating a tremendous energy. Despite the seriousness of the subject, the paintings are enlivened by a subtle playfulness.

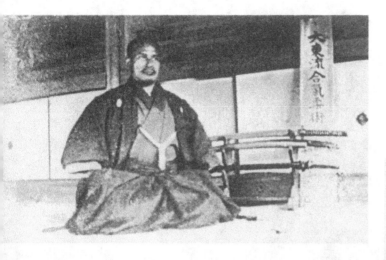

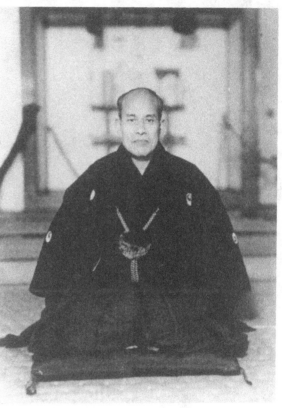

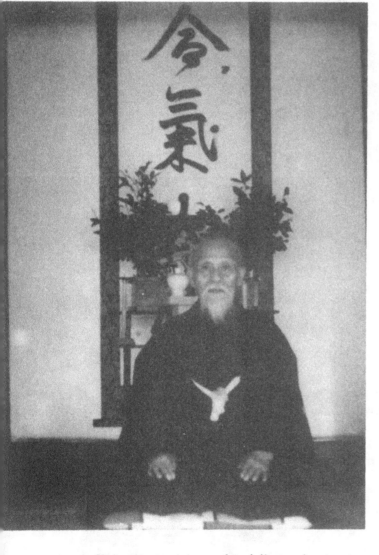

Ki is never static, and it follows changes in one's disposition. *Top:* Shown here in his intense thirties, Morihei manifests an aggressive type of *ki*, spewing forth from his *ara-mitama*. *Right:* In his fifties, Morihei's aura projects a more polished and refined *ki*. *Bottom:* In his later years, Morihei's *ki* is unsullied and bright, radiating from his *nigi-mitama*.

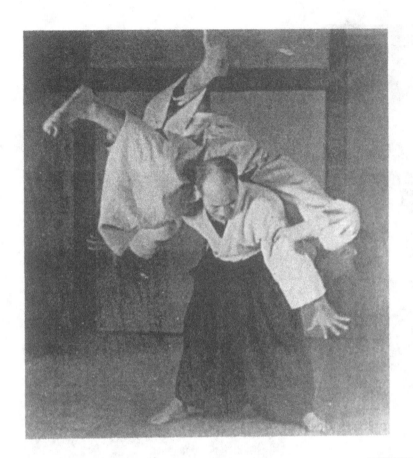

Ki permeates every portion of Morihei's body and flows from his fingertips as he executes *koshi-nage*.

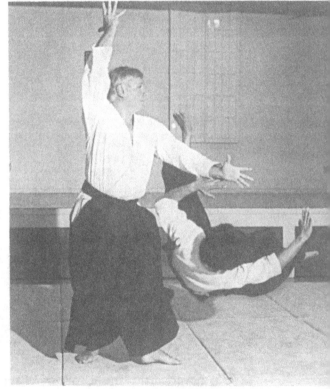

The author performing the same technique. Note that the body of the *uke*, too, is charged with *ki*, allowing him to take a breakfall without fear of injury. In this manner, both partners get to polish *ki* in each Aikidō exercise. In Aikidō, we always rely on the life force rather than on brute force and raw strength.

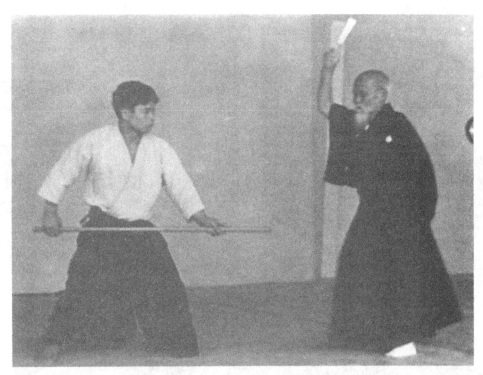

Utilizing his *ki* sensitivity, Morihei could instantaneously discern the direction of an opponent's attack and smoothly neutralize it.

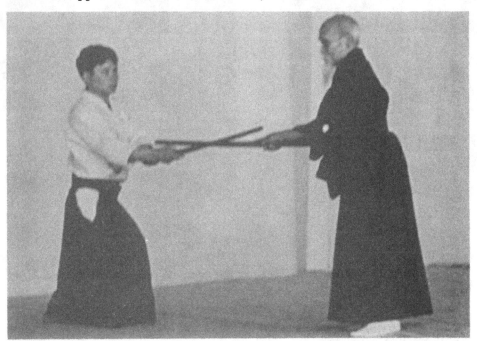

Morihei called the paired-sword exercises of Aikidō *ki-no-musubi*. That is, first you must link yourself through *ki* to your partner's striking sword, and then you must bind it with your *ki* to put a stop to the attack. It is said that at least ten years of training in such exercises are required to develop good *ki* timing.

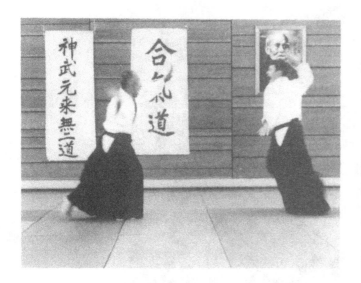

1

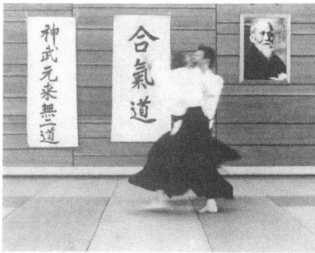

2

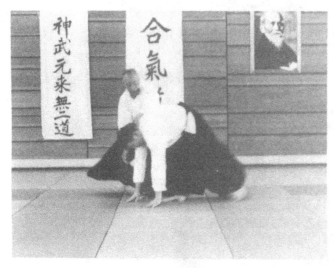

5

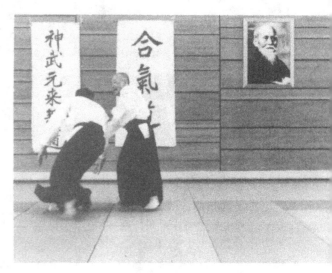

6

Ki-no-nagare, the "flow of *ki*," lies at the heart of Aikidō techniques. Here Shirata Sensei, seventy years old at the time, handles an attack by me in true Aikidō fashion, neutralizing the *ki* of the aggressive force (1, 2, 3), redirecting the *ki* flow (4, 5, 6), and then bringing the *ki* back to earth (7, 8). (In #8, I've rolled right out of the picture.)

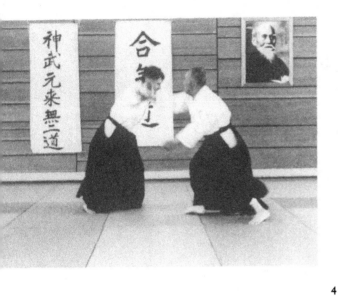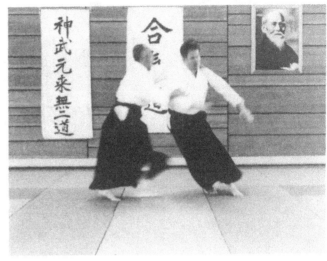

4

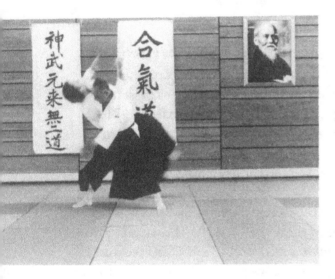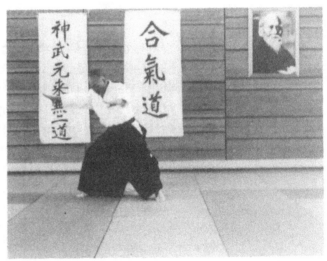

8

KOKYŪ
THE BREATH OF LIFE

WHILE *KOKYŪ* IS INEXTRICABLY BOUND WITH *KI*, IT IS FELT
that there is a subtle distinction between the two forces. *Kokyū* is just
as difficult to define as *ki*, so those distinctions cannot be neatly stated.
Kokyū is first of all "breath," the physical act of inhaling and exhaling. This
breath is the basic fact of our existence—"In the beginning was the Word"
may also be stated as "In the beginning was the Breath"—without which we
will surely expire. (There is a theory in Shintō that human beings exhale at
the time of birth and inhale at death.)

In India, breath is known as *prāṇa*. The in-breath creates the seed-syllable
HĀṂ ("I"), and the out-breath the seed-syllable SA ("this"). The natural act
of breathing produces the continual *mantra* of HĀṂSA, "I am This!"—divine
life itself. Breath is thus a natural and spontaneous prayer, a *mantra*, according to tantric texts, that is repeated 21,600 times a day. In Japanese esoteri-
cism, the out-breath is *haku*, masculine, and the in-breath is *su*, feminine. In
each cycle of our breath we have the natural harmonization of male and female, fire and water, and the formation of *ka-mi*.

Kokyū, like *ki*, is thought of as a pervasive cosmic force: "Breath is the
thread that ties creation together." The entire universe is breathing—high tide
marks the peak of the cosmic inhalation, and low tide means that the cosmic
exhalation is complete. Izanagi and Izanami are actually still alive, bound
tightly together; Izanagi takes one full breath every 182½ days from midwinter to midsummer, and Izanami takes her breath for the following 182½ days
from midsummer to midwinter.

Morihei encouraged each student to link his or her individual breath to the cosmic breath:

> Consider the ebb and flow of the tide. When waves come to strike the shore, they crest and fall, creating a sound. Your breath should follow the same pattern, absorbing the entire universe in your belly with each inhalation. Know that we all have access to four treasures: the energy of the sun and moon, the breath of heaven, the breath of earth, and the ebb and flow of the tide.

Technically, *kokyū* means "concentrated power," and "good timing." *Kokyū* is the dynamo that sustains accomplished masters—allowing a musician to hold endlessly long notes, a Noh actor to move about the stage for hours in full costume, and a martial artist to deal with opponent after opponent without tiring. There is a special set of exercises in Aikidō employed to build breath power; they teach a practitioner how to breathe with the entire body and thus generate explosive vigor. (The difference here between *kiai* and *kokyū* power is not easy to explain.)

Kokyū is the good timing between an artist and his medium of expression, between master and disciple, between *uke* and *nage,* between oneself and the world. If the *kokyū* of two people, or a group, is out of synchronization, it is certain to spell trouble. The original meaning of the Hawaiian greeting "aloha" is based on this premise. *Alo* means to experience the *ha,* the "breath" or "life force" of another. That is, two people become friends by exchanging and blending their *aloha,* their *kokyū. Kokyū* is further understood as the natural rhythm that exists in all activities; to be truly successful in any endeavor, one has to be in harmony with the *kokyū* of the moment. This is the "knack" of making the right move in Aikidō and any other art.

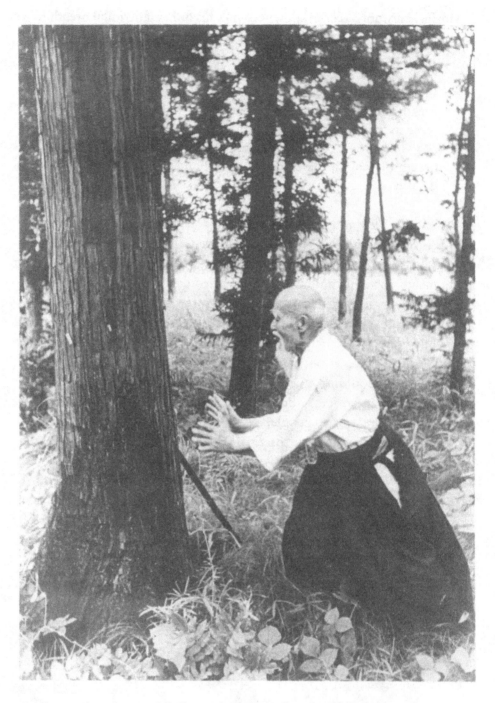

Morihei performing an Aikidō exercise outside to build *kokyū* power. Nature is an inexhaustible source of *kokyū*, and we must learn how to harness and concentrate that force.

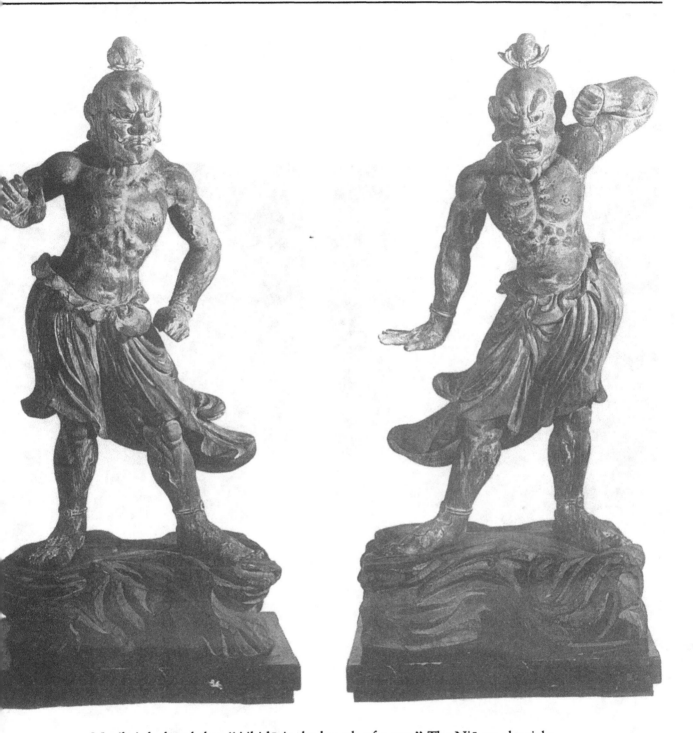

Morihei declared that "Aikidō is the breath of A-UN." The Niō on the right pronounces the A *kototama,* a shout that drives away all eternal enemies; the Niō on the left has his mouth closed in the UN *kototama,* a sign of determination to battle inner foes. A-UN is the same as Alpha-Omega, the all encompassing truth of the universe. The A-UN breath is smooth, natural, and eternally extended. Both Niō assume postures that are regularly employed in Aikidō—in *irimi* and *kaiten* throws, for example.

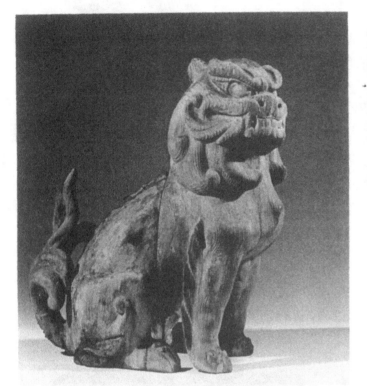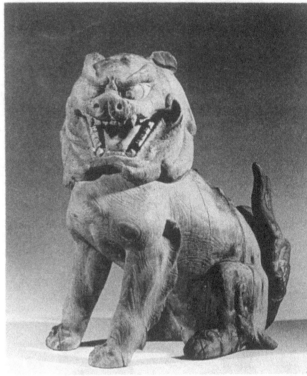

In Shintō, the A-UN *kokyū* is represented by two shrine guardian dogs. The
animal powers, too, can teach us valuable lessons.

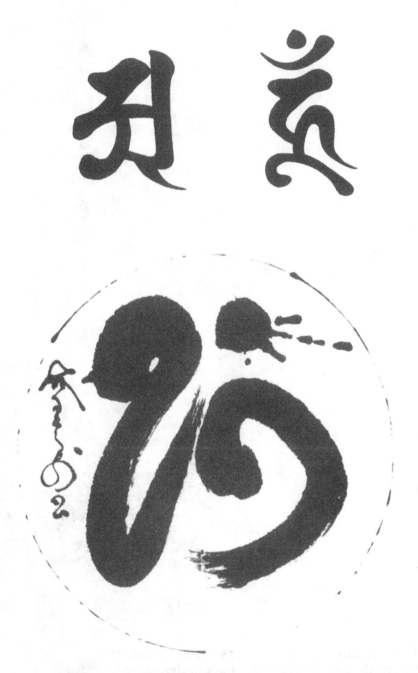

Top: A and UN (pronounced HŪM in Sanskrit) written in Siddham script. A is the seed-syllable of the Womb Matrix, while HŪM is that of the Diamond Matrix. Pronounced together, the two sounds encompass the universe.

Bottom: The Chinese character for the seed-syllable A written in cursive style by Tesshū Yamaoka (1836–1888). This calligraphy is pure *kokyū*.

"The Noh Dancer," Zen painting by Shunsō (1750–1839). Good *kokyū* is indispensable for the performance arts. In Noh drama, for instance, the actor must be perfectly attuned to the musicians and the audience for the production to be a success. Zeami, the father of Noh theater, once told his students: "A Noh actor must be at his best when the audience is at its worst." That is, only a scintillating performance, overflowing with breath power, can lift a listless and inattentive audience out of its stupor. Incidentally, the dance movement the actor displays here is very similar to the *ippon-ashi* movement of *aiki* sword play.

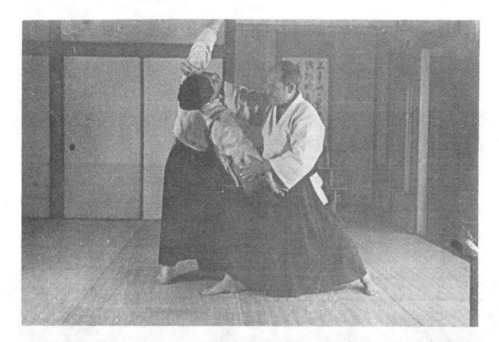

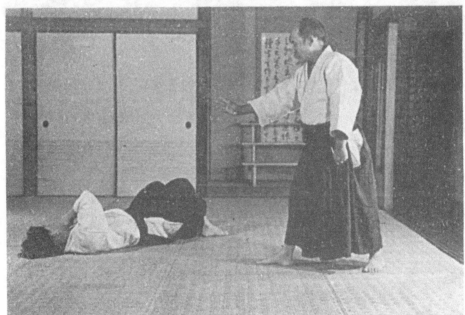

Morihei demonstrating a *kokyū* throw. Such a technique relies on perfect timing, what the great swordsman Musashi described as "striking down an opponent in a single beat."

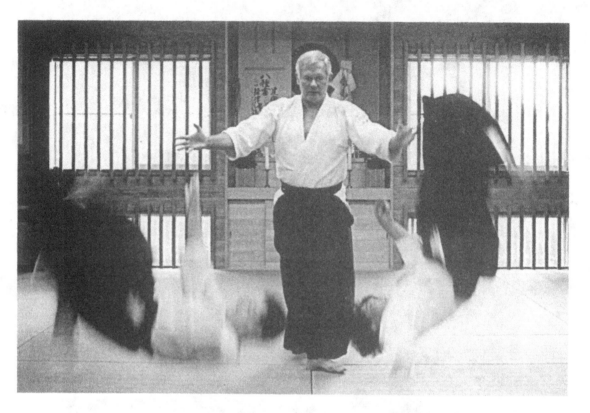

Kokyū: Stillness in the midst of movement.

CHINKON-KISHIN
CALMING THE SPIRIT, RETURNING TO THE SOURCE

*C*HINKON MEANS "SETTLE DOWN AND CALM THE SPIRIT." THIS is a common approach to religious practice everywhere. Daily life is full of distractions, and most people find their physical and psychic energy quickly dispersed and expended on external affairs, large and small. Human beings regularly need to pull themselves together through some form of quiet meditation.

For his *chinkon,* Morihei relied on traditional Shintō methods:

1. *Tori-fune* (*kōgi-fune undō*), "rowing the boat" (punctuated with *kototama* yells like ES-SA, ES-SA). This continues to be a popular exercise in many Aikidō *dōjō.* It combines good training for body stability as well as helping to concentrate the mind.

2. *Otakebi,* "valorous shout of victory," somewhat akin to the cheer "hip, hip, hurray!" Typically, *otakebi* included the *kototama* shouts IKU-TAMA, TARU-TAMA, and TAMA-TOMARU-TAMA, followed by the calling out of the name of a Shintō deity.

3. *Okorobi,* "rite of purification," in which one forms the "spear *mudrā*" with the right hand and cuts down with a sharp *kiai* to drive away all demons in the vicinity.

4. *Ibuki,* "deep breathing of the body," and *furitama,* "vibration of the spirit." The deep breathing exercises take a variety of forms (one type can be seen in the dedication ceremony performed by Grand Champion sumō wrestlers). In *furitama* the hands are

clasped tightly together in front of one's *tanden* and then shaken up and down to calm the spirit and vibrate the soul.

Chinkon should lead into *kishin*, "returning to the *kami*," a deeper contemplative state in which one is grounded in the divine. Morihei once recommended this method:

> Sit quietly in either *seiza* or *zazen*. Close your eyes and place your hands in the cosmic *mudrā*. First contemplate the manifest realm for twenty minutes—how the world looks and feels. As you settle down, immerse yourself in the hidden realm and return to the source of things, the *kototama* SU. Remain there at the center as long as you can, perhaps forty minutes or so.

Morihei had performed these practices since childhood, and they were an integral part of his being, but he never made them obligatory for his students and in fact encouraged them to select and develop *chinkon-kishin* exercises that were appropriate for their own backgrounds and needs.* Morihei did emphasize, however, that some kind of meditation is essential for the practice of Aikidō: "If your *chinkon-kishin* is good, you can understand everything."

---

*I use the system outlined in *Aikidō: The Way of Harmony*, pp. 29–36.

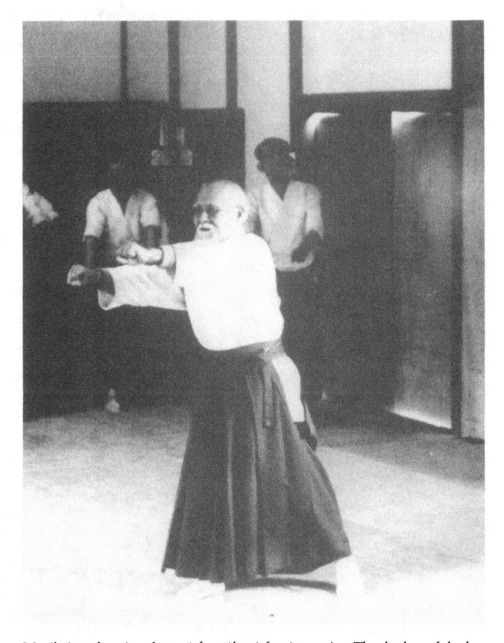

Morihei performing the *tori-fune* (*kōgi-fune*) exercise. The rhythm of the *ko-totama* rowing is: I (out) KU (in) MU (out) SU (in) BI (out). This traditional *chinkon* exercise is still widely practiced in Aikidō.

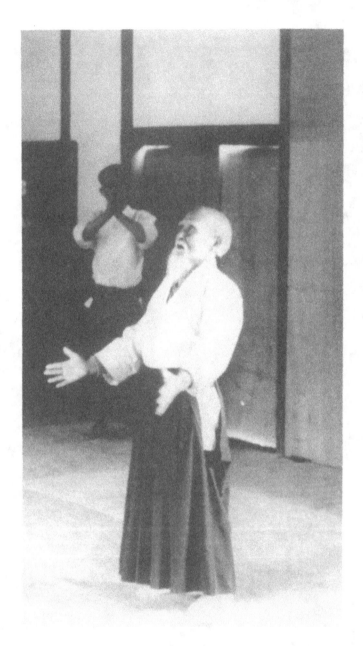

Morihei taking a deep *ibuki* breath. His physical stance here reflects a luminous and serene state of mind.

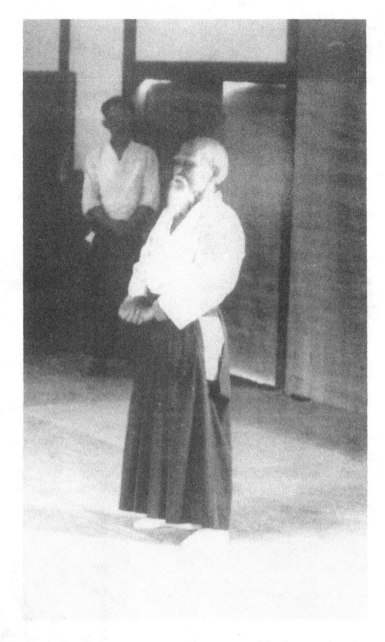

Morihei ending the *furitama* exercise in a state of *kishin*. Only after calming the spirit and returning to the source should practice of the techniques commence.

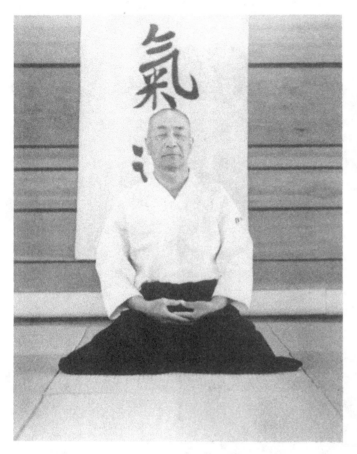

Shirata Sensei in *chinkon-kishin* with hands forming the cosmic *mudrā*. On occasion, it is valuable to practice *chinkon-kishin* individually for periods up to an hour. Morihei taught, "Always keep your mind as bright and clear as the vast sky, the great ocean, and the highest peak, empty of all thoughts."

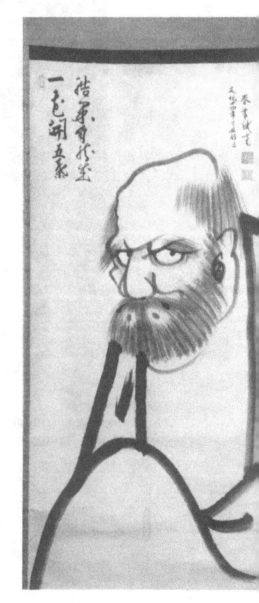

In *chinkon-kishin* the eyes are normally kept closed, but after the meditation is completed, the eyes should be as open as those of Bodhidharma, the Grand Patriarch of Zen: "One who is wide awake has no fear!" Zen painting by Shunsō (1750–1839).

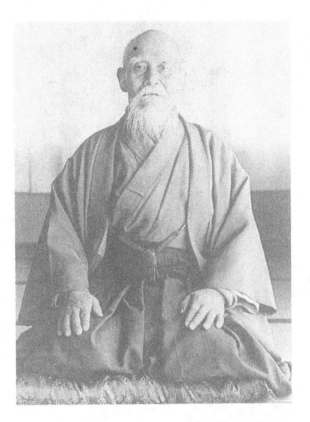

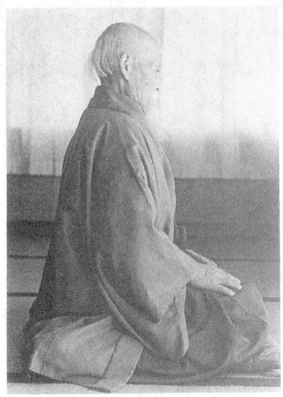

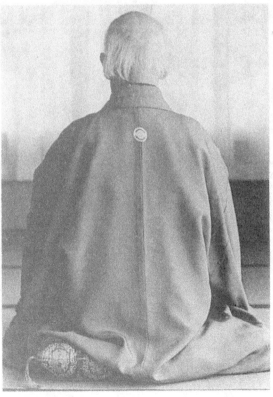

One should always strive to be "calm and close to the Source." Morihei here displays the correct form of *seiza,* which can be interpreted as "correct and serene sitting." Bodhidharma, too, is often depicted from these three angles: head-on, side view, and facing the Absolute.

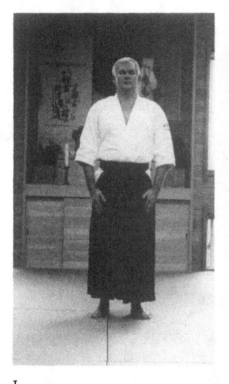

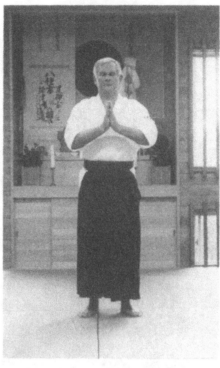

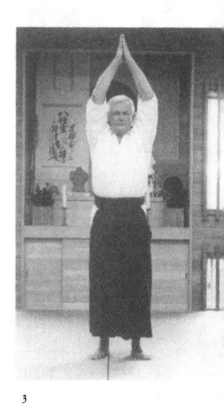

1   2   3

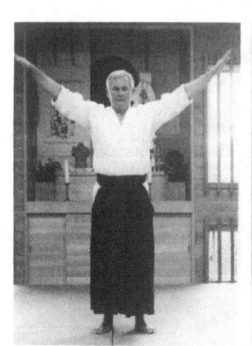

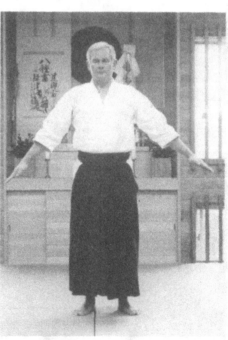

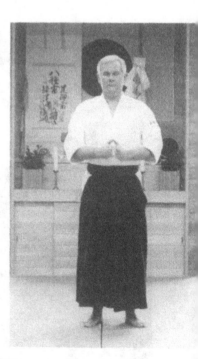

4   5   6

Ideally, practice should end as well as begin with *chinkon-kishin*. At the end of training, we perform this exercise in my *dōjō*. Inhale deeply, raising the hands in the *ten-no-kokyū* ("breath of heaven") posture (2, 3). Exhale slowly and bring the hands down in the *chi-no-kokyū* ("breath of earth") posture (4, 5, 6). Repeat three times.

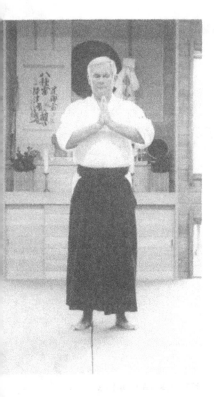
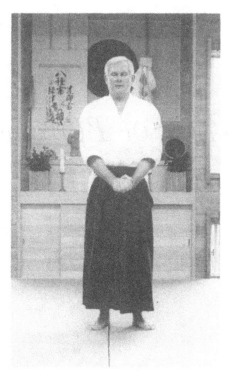
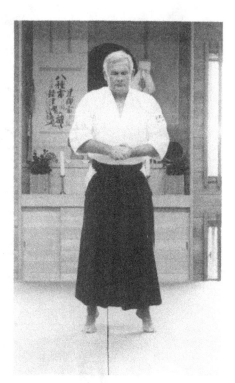

2

3

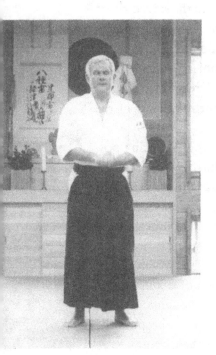
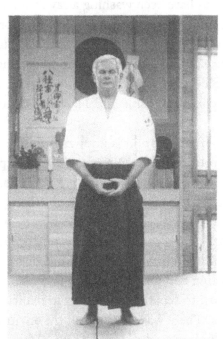

5

After completing the three heaven-and-earth breaths, perform the *furitama* exercise three times. Clasp the hands together (2), inhale right up to the top of the head, rising up naturally on the toes (3), and then exhale vigorously to the bottom of the feet, shaking the hands up and down (4). Finish with a period of silent *kishin* (5).

MISOGI
PURIFICATION OF BODY AND MIND

*P*URIFICATION WITH WATER IS YET ANOTHER UNIVERSAL RITE of religion. Hindus have been washing away their sins in the sacred rivers of India since the beginning of recorded history. Jews practice ritual immersion, Muslims perform ablutions, and Christians and Buddhists use water in their respective baptismal and *abhiṣeka* initiation ceremonies; Native Americans construct sweat lodges ("If the heart is not pure, the Great Spirit cannot be seen," said the elder Black Elk); and Hawaiians perform *hi'uwai* in the waters of the Pacific.

In Japan, this kind of purification is known as *misogi*. After suffering pollution in the dark world of the dead, Izanagi went to purify himself in the swift waters of Tachibana-no-Odo (*Kojiki* 1:11). Various deities came into being as a result of Izanagi's *misogi*, the foremost being Amaterasu and Susano-o; thus purification with water—in the ocean, under a waterfall, or from ice-cold buckets—was a central religious practice in Japan.

Cleansing the body of filth was just one kind of *misogi*, however. There was the *misogi* of fasting and proper diet to purge the body of toxins. There was *misogi* of the heart, to separate oneself from malicious thoughts, unkind words, and bad deeds. There was a *misogi* of the environment—keeping the things around oneself clean and in good order. When all these things were accomplished, *misogi* became a ritual of positive change and renewal.

Morihei engaged in all these traditional *misogi* rites but finally concluded that Aikidō itself is one all-inclusive form of *misogi*: "The essence of Aikidō is to cleanse yourself of maliciousness, to get in tune with your environment, and to clear your path of all obstacles and barriers."

Morihei often quoted a stanza he had learned when he was studying the Hōzōin art of the spear: "The Way consists above all of setting your own heart aright; after that, you can face any foe certain of victory." Indeed, for Morihei, *misogi* and Aikidō became synonymous, "a cleansing of the body and soul, a radiant state of unadorned purity, an accomplishment of true harmony, a vibrant state of grace."

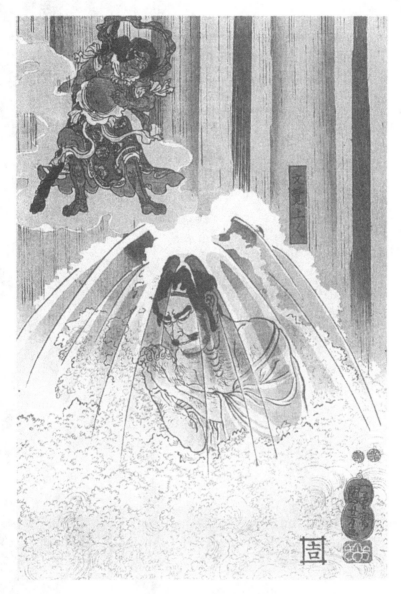

he Buddhist monk Mongaku undergoing *misogi* in the Nachi Falls (Woodblock print by Utagawa Kuniyoshi, 797–1864.) According to the *Heike Monogatari,* Mongaku made a vow to remain in *misogi* beneath the falls r thirty-seven straight days. Within a week, however, Mongaku lost consciousness, and he was washed down-ream. Two youthful attendant gods, one male and one female, rescued him by reviving the ascetic with their arm, scented hands. Thus recovered, Mongaku returned to the falls to complete his *misogi.* The Nachi Falls in umano is perhaps the best place in Japan for *misogi,* and in his early days Morihei often trained there.

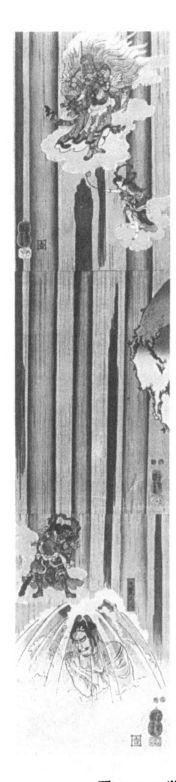
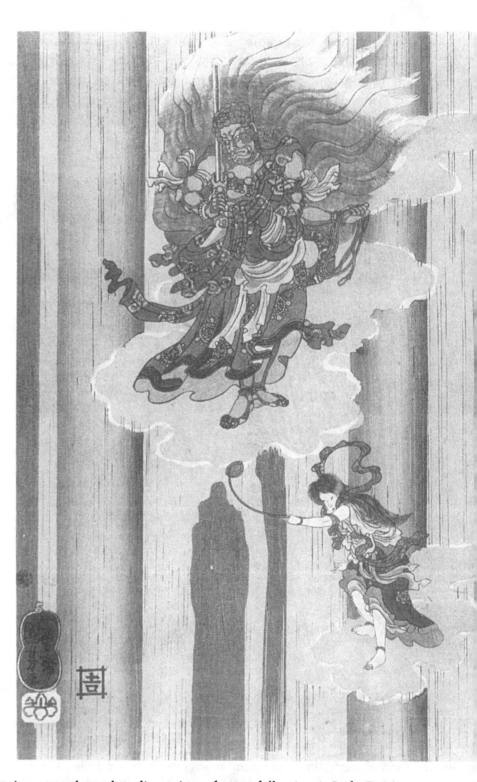

These two illustrations reveal another dimension of waterfall *misogi. Left:* Deities often manifest themselves to the ascetic. In this case, Fudō Myō-ō (*top,* with two attendant gods beneath appear to Mongaku. *Right:* Fudō Myō-ō, the Buddhist counterpart of Ame-no-Tajikara-o, is one of the patron saints of Aikidō, a symbol of fierce determination and unshakable presence of mind.

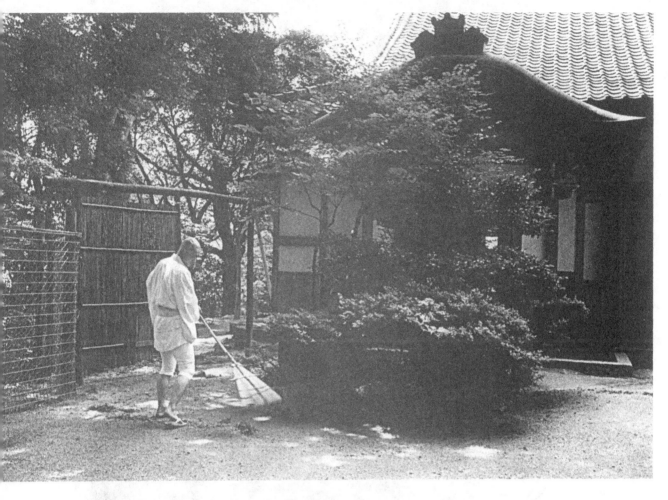

Misogi of the environment is also essential, especially important in the modern world. Zen *misogi* stresses sweeping and mopping, and the motto of some temples is: "Cleaning first; sūtra chanting second; and book learning third."

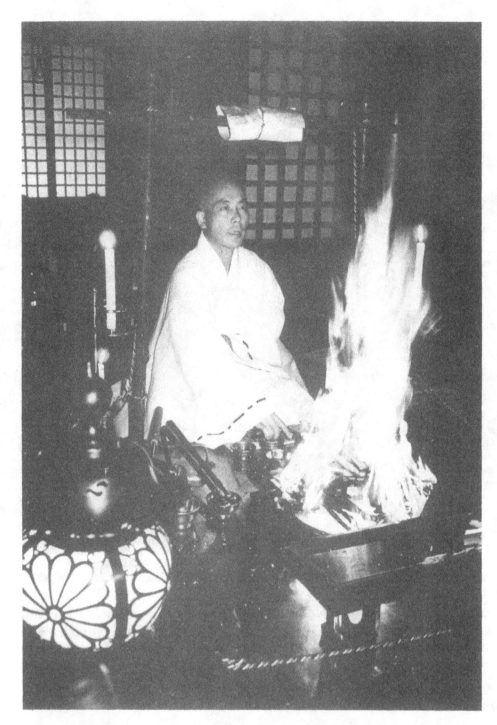

Marathon monk Shunsō Utsumi performing the Tendai Fire Ceremony. *Misogi* can be accomplished by fire as well as by water. Defiling passions, and unwholesome thoughts should be confined to the flames, and the alchemical fire can assist us in forging base matter into gold. Morihei stated: "Free the six senses from obstruction, and your entire body and soul will glow."

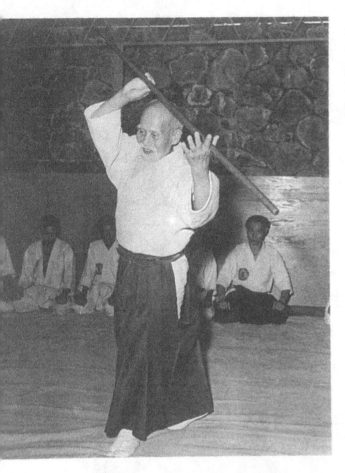

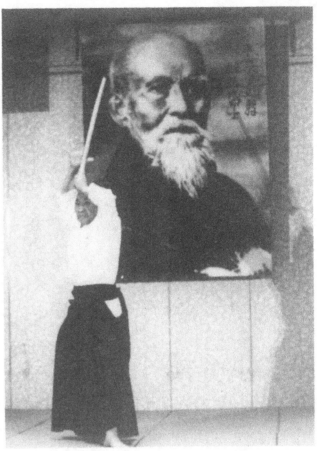

Left: A staff becomes a magic wand when wielded by sages and seers. Moses bore the "staff of God" that allowed him to part the Red Sea and bring forth water from the desert rocks (Exodus 14:16 and 17:6); Christian bishops carry crosiers as a symbol of the church's majesty; Śiva's trident is always at hand, and his Hindu devotees travel the land with their sturdy *danda;* and Taoist immortals use their sacred sticks as vehicles to manifest the mysteries of *yin* and *yang.* In Aikidō, we have *misogi-no-jō,* the "staff of purification." Morihei did *misogi-no-jō* to prepare himself for each training session. In his *misogi-no-jō* (which differed each time) Morihei spanned the four directions, heaven and earth, and three realms of manifest, hidden, and divine.

Right: The sword, too, is an instrument of purification cutting right to the heart of things, severing all doubt and confusion. In many religious sects in Japan there is a rite called *bokken-kaji,* in which a wooden sword is used to dispel all evil. Here Shirata Sensei performs *misogi-no-ken* at a memorial demonstration for the Founder.

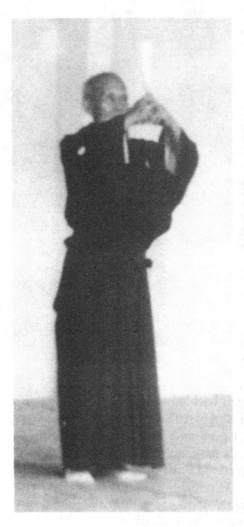 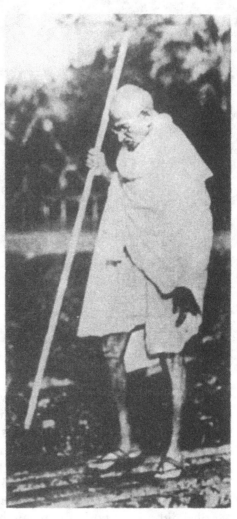

Left: On occasion, Morihei performed *misogi* movements with a fan. He defined *tsumi* (sin) as "ignorance of the universal, timeless principles of existence. Such ignorance is a floodgate for evil behavior." *Right:* Gandhi carrying his *misogi-no-jo*. The Indian *mahatma's* message was similiar to that of Morihei: "Nonviolence is impossible without self-purification."

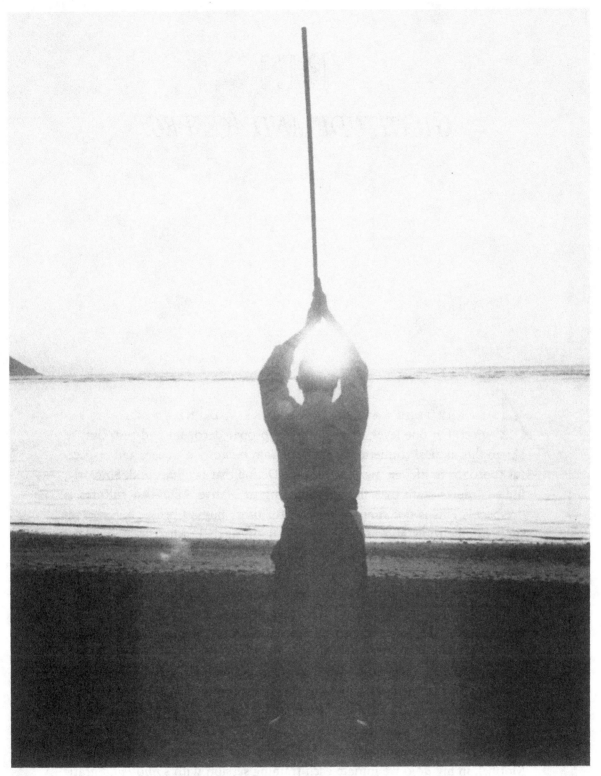

The sun is a powerful agent of *misogi*. Morihei sang:

> *The Divine Light*
> *that spans Heaven*
> *must descend to Earth*
> *and illuminate everything*
> *right to the bottom of the sea.*

REI
GRATITUDE AND RESPECT

*A*s in any true art, Aikidō begins and ends with *REI*, respect. On one level, respect implies proper decorum and restraint. In
Shintō this natural etiquette should flow from *makoto*, a sincere and respect-
ful approach to life, an awareness of the Divine that is all around. Similarly,
Indian leaders state that the underpinning of Native American cultures is
"respect." This is not simply a respect for other human beings but also respect for the tools and utensils we rely upon in daily life, the animal and
plant food we eat, and the sun, air, and water that sustain us.

When the traditional craftsmen of Japan acquired a new tool, it was not
put into use until it had been properly dedicated. Many tools were given
names, emphasizing the fact that the instrument was now part of the craftsman's family. On New Year's Day, the craftsman would lovingly clean and
polish his tools and present them with festive rice cakes. When a tool was
finally worn out, it was not simply discarded but formally retired in a special
ceremony to commemorate its long and faithful service. In Aikidō, we feel
that the *jo* and *ken* are our tools. If not handled properly, neither instrument
will respond in the right manner.

Respect is expressed by a sense of gratitude. Following the example of
Morihei, in my *dōjō* we initiate each training session with *shihō-hai*, "gratitude in the four directions." This gratitude is also a heartfelt prayer, a deep
sense of reverence for the Path and the Way of Aikidō.

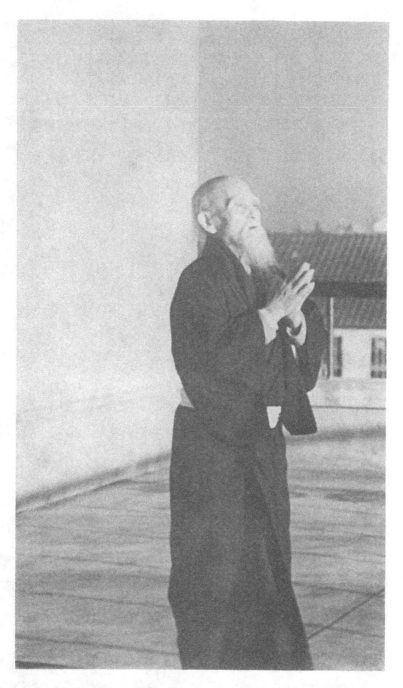

Morihei pays his respect to the rising sun. Even when he was staying in the center of busy, noisy, crowded Tokyo, Morihei would climb to the roof of the Hombu Dōjō at daybreak to offer his salutations to the sun. The attitude of *gasshō,* with the hands clasped in prayer, is often said to be the most beautiful a human being can assume. The left hand represents the sun, fire, the Diamond Matrix; the right hand stands for the moon, water, the Womb Matrix. In Buddhism, the praying hands posture is called the "*mudrā* of unshakable sincerity."

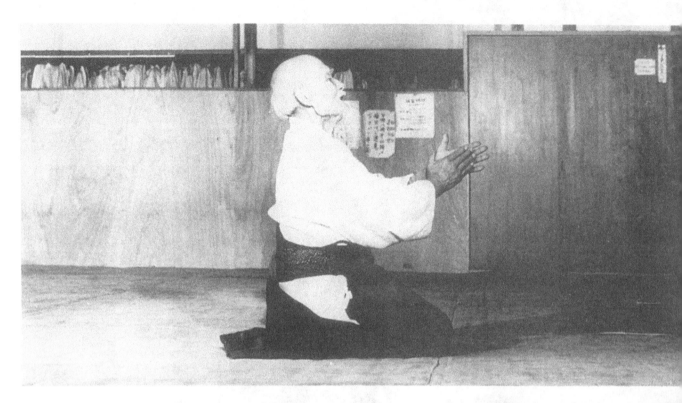

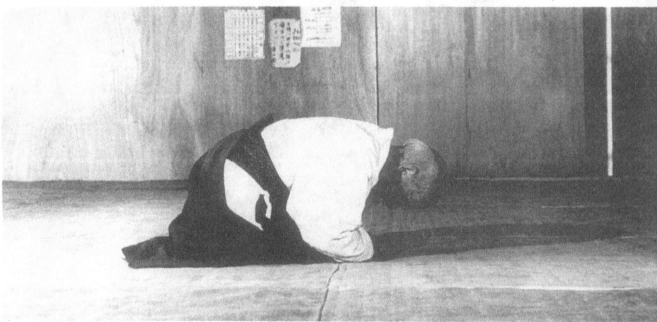

Morihei bowing to the *dōjō* shrine at the beginning of practice. Aikidō begins and ends wit *rei*. The Aikidō bow is not the suspicious and cautious greeting one makes to a potential fo but a deep and genuine genuflection all the way to the ground. Sometimes a bow is accom panied with the clapping of hands to announce one's presence to the gods. Once Morihei pai a visit to a disciple's *dōjō* and bowed to the shrine. Morihei then suddenly turned to h student and said sharply, "You did not greet the *kamisama* this morning!" "Yes," the discip admitted sheepishly, "I was so busy preparing for your visit, I neglected my morning prayers. "Never forget to pay your respects!" Morihei scolded him. "That is what Aikidō is all about.

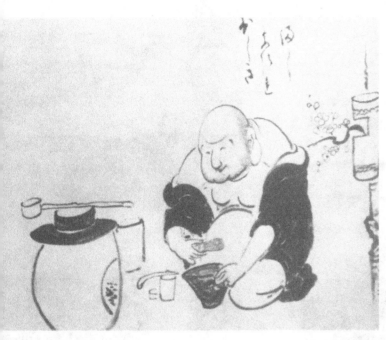

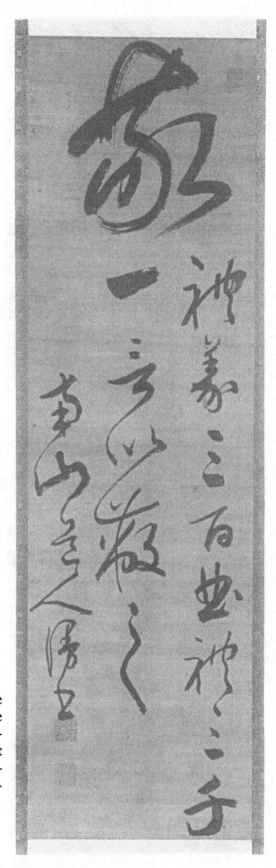

en painting of Hotei preparing tea, by Hakuin (1685–1768).
Honor and respect is a cardinal tenet of the tea ceremony, too.
ne has to learn how to care for and handle both the utensils
nd one's guests. After the prescribed procedures are mastered,
natural etiquette should emerge in which the taste of tea and
en are one.

Respect (*kei*)—There are three hundred Shintō rules and three
ousand Confucian codes, but all of them are based on this one
ord," brushed by the Zen monk Nanzan (1756–1839). The es-
nce of Shintō, Confucian, and Buddhist ethics is respect—respect
r gods and buddhas, respect for physical objects, respect for hu-
an beings. Respect is not simply consideration; it includes identi-
cation with, and sympathy for, another's position.

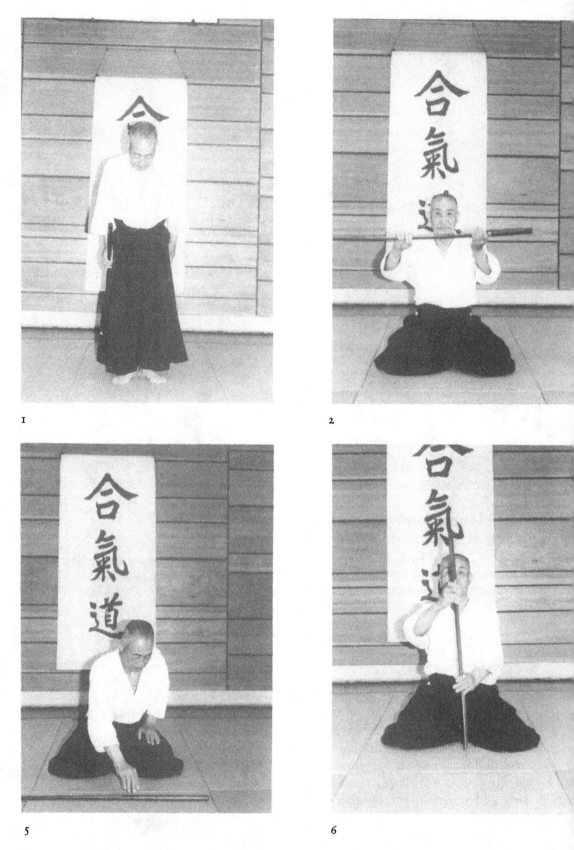

1

2

5

6

Shirata Sensei demonstrates the proper Aikidō etiquette for handling the sword. The sword
not an instrument of destruction, but a sacred implement of purification and transformatio

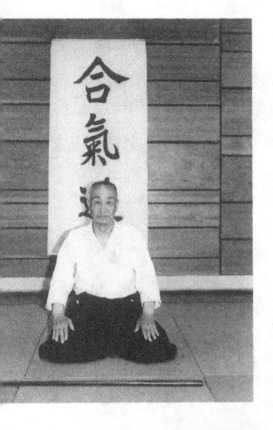

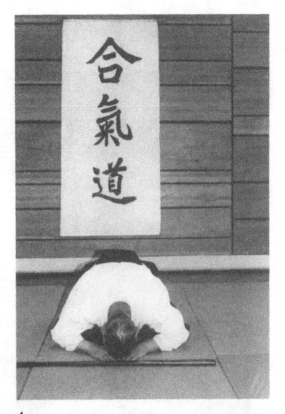

4

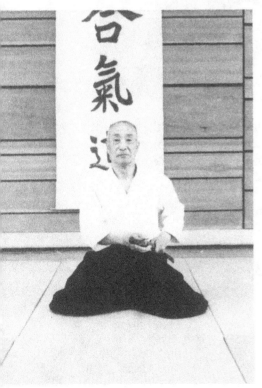

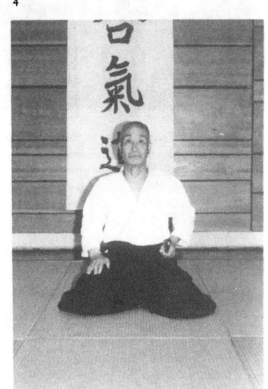

8

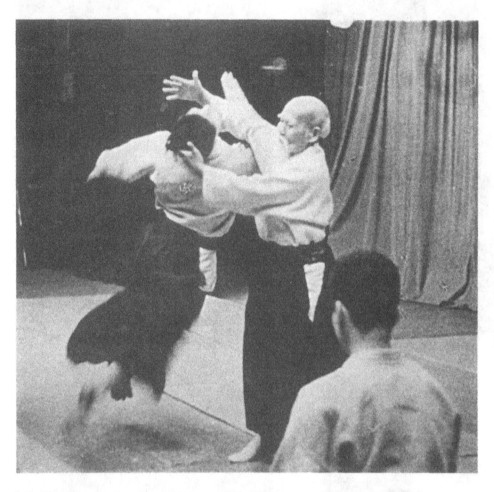

Morihei taught that in Aikidō we should treat our partner with the utmost respect. One's partner is entrusting his or her life to you, and we must handle that precious object with the greatest care. Morihei often counseled his students, "Hold your partner as you would cradle a baby."

SANGEN
TRIANGLE, CIRCLE, AND SQUARE

MORIHEI OFTEN REMARKED, "THE ONLY WAY I CAN REALLY explain Aikidō is to draw a triangle, circle, and square"—the three most perfect proportions of geometry.

A triangle with its point ascending symbolizes fire and the cosmic *liṇga*; with its point descending, it stands for water and the cosmic *yoni*. The three sides of the triangle represent various trinities: heaven, earth, and humankind; mind, body, and spirit; past, present, and future. A triangle signifies the dimension of *ki* flow.

A circle is a universal emblem for infinity, perfection, and eternity. Nature expresses itself in circles, circuits, and spirals. A circle is zero, the emptiness that fulfills all things. It represents the liquid dimension.

A square is stable, orderly, and material. It is the base of the physical world, composed of earth, water, fire, and air. The square signifies the solid dimension.

It is also important to conceive of the *sangen* in their three-dimensional forms: tetrahedron (pyramid), sphere, and cube. Morihei said about the three fundamentals:

The triangle represents the generation of energy and initiative; it is the most stable physical posture. The circle symbolizes unification, serenity, and perfection; it is the source of unlimited techniques. The square stands for form and solidity, the basis of applied control.

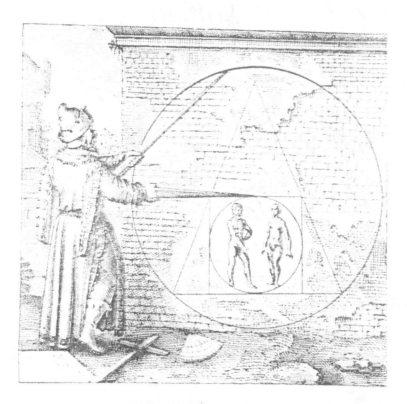

Diagram from an eighteenth-century alchemical text: "From a man and woman create circle, a square, a triangle, and then another circle and you will thus obtain the Philosopher's Stone."

Another Western alchemical diagram. The same configuration of circle, triangle, and square is commonly seen adorning Aikidō *dōjō*. The esoteric significance of the sun-fire-king and moon-water-queen symbols is also familiar to students of Aikidō.

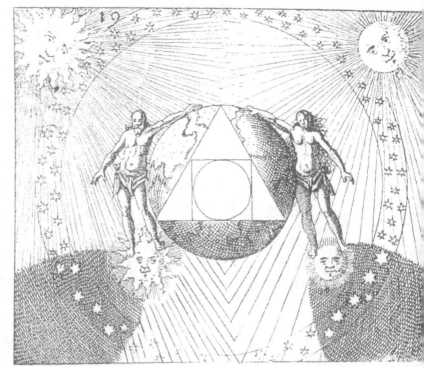

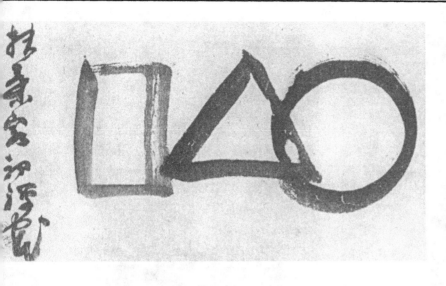

"Circle, Triangle, Square" by Sengai (1750–1838). This image can be interpreted on many levels, but for Aikidō students the explanation that most readily comes to mind is the integration of heaven (circle), humankind (triangle), and earth (square).

Triangle, circle, and square symbolism in a Tibetan *maṇḍala*. The *liṅga* and *yoni* triangles intersect (as in the Seal of Solomon), representing the fusing of the Diamond and Womb Matrixes. The Three Fundamentals give structure and stability to the universe, a truth we should always be cognizant of during Aikidō training.

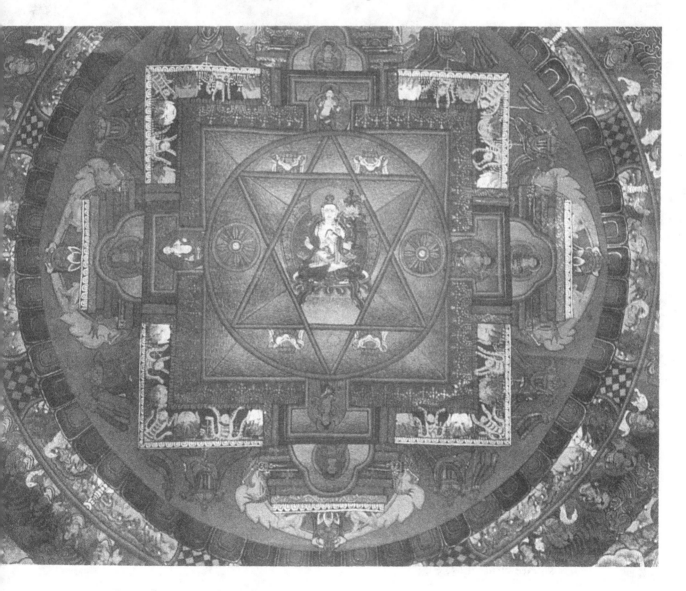

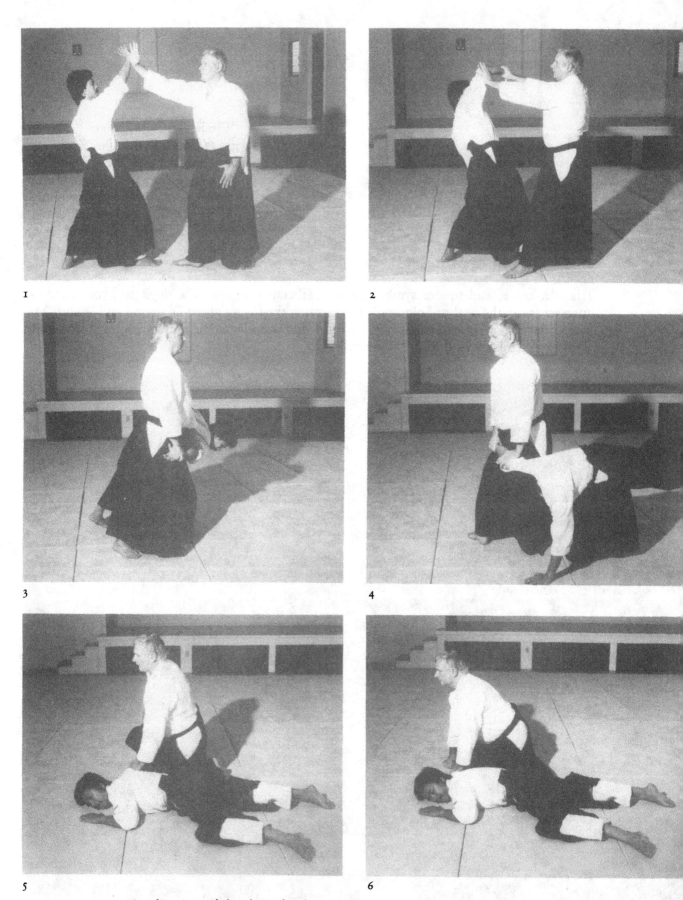

Application of the three fundamentals: triangular entry (1, 2); circular blending (3, 4); ar square control (5, 6).

MA-AI
THE RIGHT PLACE

ONE OF THE DISTINCTIVE FEATURES OF ASIAN CULTURE IS MA, which can mean, depending on the circumstance, "room," "space," "interval," "timing," or "rhythm." In painting, extensive use is made of *ma* as negative space. That is, large sections of the painting are left blank or very vaguely brushed to suggest clouds, distant mountains, vast bodies of water, and the like. In calligraphy, spacing is even more critical, and the mark of a true artist is the ability to naturally place a character in just the right spot.

Ma is also exhibited in music, dance, drama, comedy, and literature. This *ma* is in the realm of intuition and timing, and it is a kind of three-dimensional *kokyū*. To use the example of Noh drama, the musical accompanists frequently let out energizing shouts at exactly the right moment between the choppy intervals in the actor's lines. Such shouts, of course, cannot be written into the score—they have to be emitted spontaneously. *Ma* is as crucial to the success of the performing arts as *kokyū*—a contemporary Japanese comedian in fact killed himself because he had lost his "sense of *ma*." One reason Japanese poetry is so short—only seventeen syllables in the case of *haiku*—is that it is up to the reader to enter into the *ma* space between each word and phrase to discern the poet's intention.

Ma-ai is critical in *budō*. Too far away from the opponent, it is impossible to strike or counter; too close and one is hemmed in. In the classical martial arts, it is always the teacher or senior disciple who receives the attacking force first because a beginning student cannot be expected to adjust his or her *ma-ai* immediately.

On a broader level, *ma-ai* means to appreciate another's space, to learn how to adjust to various conditions, and to develop a good sense of timing in human affairs—just what Aikidō is all about.

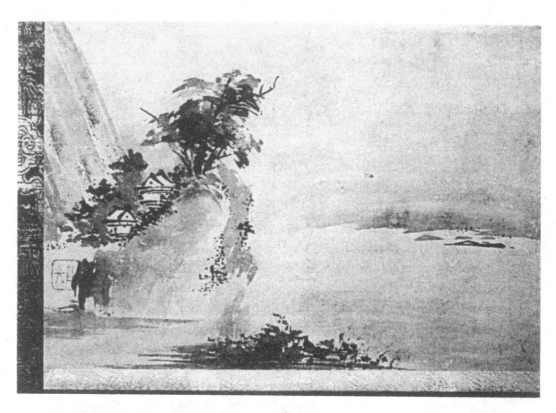

Ma spacing in a Zen painting attributed to Miyamoto Musashi (1584–1645). The work bristles with energy, and the cliffs to the left are set off against the islands to the right with a perfect sense of *ma-ai*.

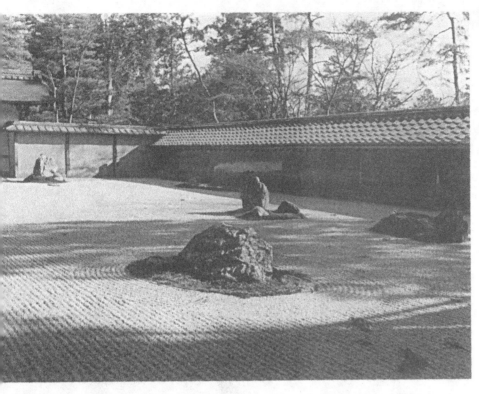

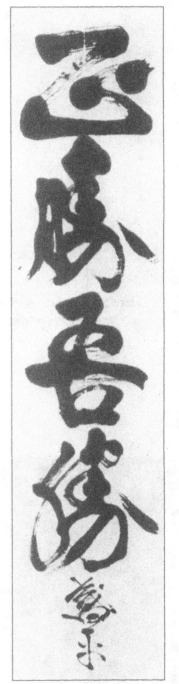

The placement of the rocks in the famous garden of Ryōan-ji in Kyōtō displays wonderful *ma* spacing. One gets the feeling that the rocks are in no way static entities—there is a vital flow of energy all through this garden.

Morihei's *aiki ma-ai* is clearly evident in his calligraphy of *Masakatsu Agatsu*. The flow of the brush, the spacing of the characters, and the decisive finish all attest to a vibrant sense of *ma-ai*.

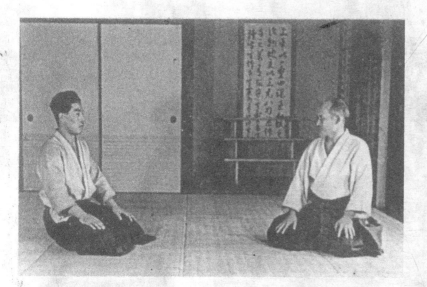

Morihei demonstrates the proper *ma-ai* fo
seated techniques. This old-fashioned
dōjō, too, is laid out in strict accordance
to the dictates of *ma*.

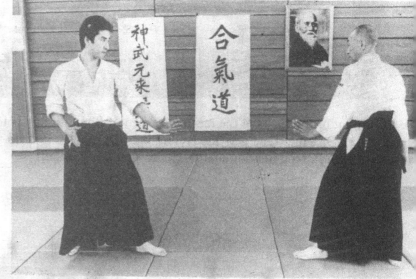

Here Shirata Sensei displays proper
ma-ai for standing techniques.

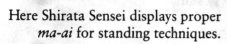

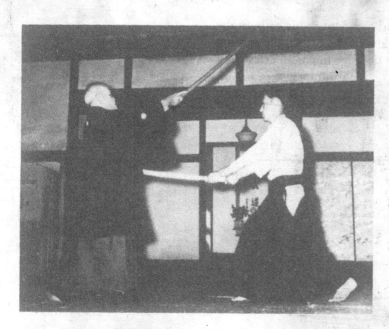

Morihei, shown here with his son Kisshomaru,
taught that training in *aiki-ken* fosters both
good timing and good spacing.

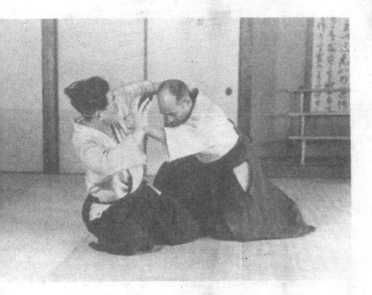

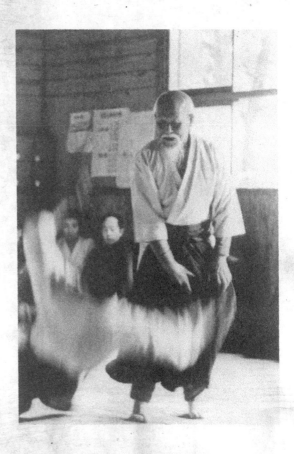

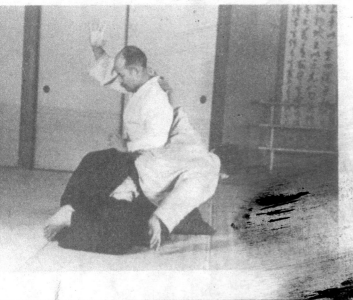

Zanshin, "retention of the mind," is another function of *ma.* As seen in the conclusion of the technique shown here (3), Morihei remains in contact with his partner even though he is not physically touching *uke.* Morihei's concentration is unbroken, and he is in the position of being able to respond to any contingency. In the illustration above, Morihei's *zanshin* is more relaxed but just as strong and stable. In his later years, Morihei's *ma-ai* sense was so refined that he barely had to touch his partners to bring them down.

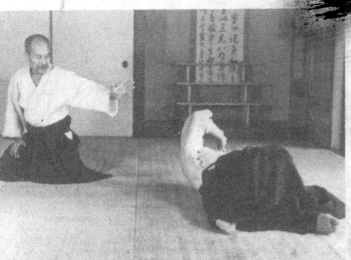

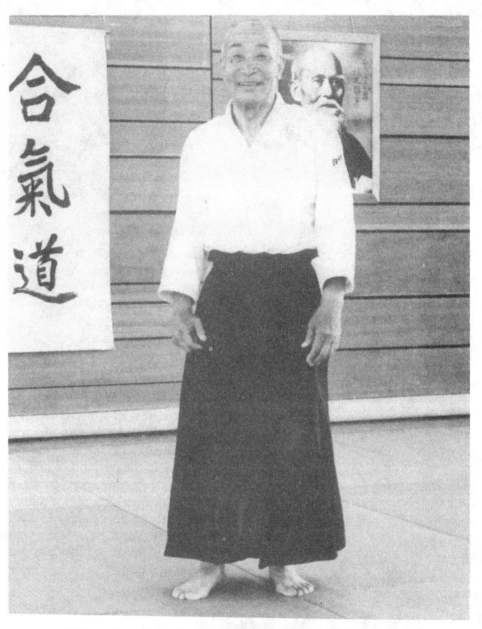

Shirata Sensei displaying the best kind of Aikidō *zanshin*.

TENGU
THE MASTER TEACHERS

MORIHEI LOVED THE FOLLOWING TALE:

Ushiwaka-maru's father, Yoshitomo, the head of the Minamoto clan, had been killed when his army had been routed by that of the Taira clan. Ushiwaka-maru's life was spared, but at the age of seven he was sent to a temple on Mount Kurama, near Kyōtō, to be raised by Buddhist monks and kept out of mischief. The young novice, however, had but one thought: "I must avenge the death of my father!" Ushiwaka-maru began sneaking out of the temple at night to practice fencing in spooky Shōjō Valley, a ravine so thick with pine and cedar that the sunlight could barely penetrate the trees even in midday. Imagining the thick trunks of the forest to be Taira troops, Ushiwaka-maru whacked away at them all night with a sword fashioned from a branch.

One evening a strange-looking *yamabushi* emerged from the gloom and offered to initiate the lad into the secrets of swordsmanship. Fearless, Ushiwaka-maru yelled, "Let's start right now!" and lashed out at the wild-looking monk. After failing to strike a single blow, Ushiwaka-maru begged the *yamabushi* to teach him. Each night thereafter, the boy took lessons with the the master Shōjō-bō and his band of *tengu*. By the age of twelve, Ushiwaka-maru could hold his own with even the most powerful *tengu*—he was now ready to leave the mountain. Ushiwaka-maru went on to defeat the Herculean monk Benkei in an epic battle, emerging as one of Japan's greatest warriors, and it is said that in the following centuries every great martial artist followed his example by learning swordsmanship from the *tengu*.

Morihei, too, secluded himself on Mount Kurama and often spoke of the *tengu* who came to cross swords with him. Disciples who accompanied Morihei on some of the training sessions conducted on Mount Kurama relate that it frequently seemed as if Morihei were battling an army of invisible foes. And in certain of the films that remain of Morihei, it appears that he is sparring with an opponent that others cannot clearly see. (This is particularly true of a film shot in Hawaii at the dedication of the Honolulu *dōjō*—perhaps Morihei is pacifying the local Hawaiian *tengu*.) Morihei firmly believed in the reality of *tengu* and other inhabitants of the spirit world. The existence of such manifestations cannot be explained rationally, so it is best to think of them as "Mysterious Secrets of the Mind."

Tantric practice relies on "Three Mysterious Secrets: of the Body, of Speech, and of the Mind." In the idiom of Aikidō, the physical techniques constitute the secrets of the Body, and *kototama* express the secrets of Speech. Secrets of the Mind are based on visualizations and subsequent projections. That is, one focuses initially on an image of a god or a buddha and attempts to attain union with the object of contemplation. Profound visualization spontaneously leads to projection, an actualization of the image—for example, a *tengu*—within one's own mind *and* in three dimensions. As Tantric philosophers say, "One becomes that which one thinks of constantly." (This kind of three-dimensional projection is the source of all iconography.) Since "everything within is everything without" in Tantra, the potentialities inside a human being correspond to potentialities in the "outside" world. But because both our outer and inner vision is muddled, we fail to perceive the gods (and demons) that circulate within and all about us. One of the purposes of *chinkon-kishin* and *misogi* is to restore our pure vision—then perhaps the *tengu* will come and teach us, too.

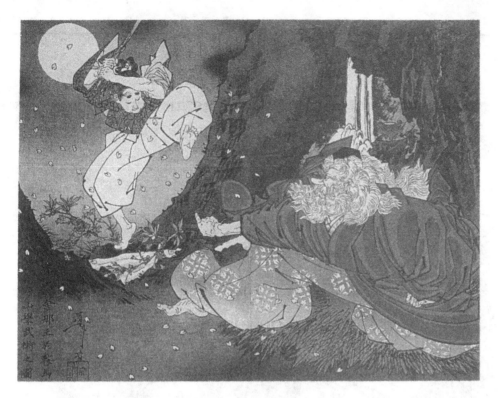

Shōjō-bō, the Tengu King, imparts the secrets of the sword to Ushiwaka-maru on Mount Kurama in this print by Tsukioka Yoshitoshi (1839–1892). This is an extremely popular theme in Japanese art and literature.

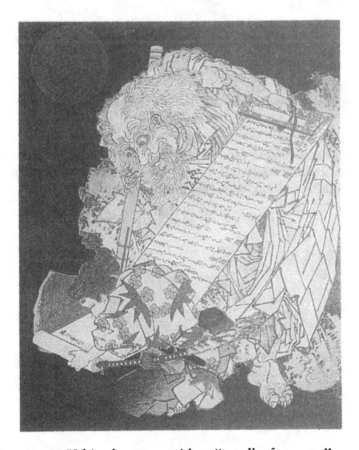

Shōjō-bō presents Ushiwaka-maru with a "scroll of secrets," consisting of *dōka,* "Songs of the Way." Woodblock print by Yanagawa Shigenobu (1787–1852).

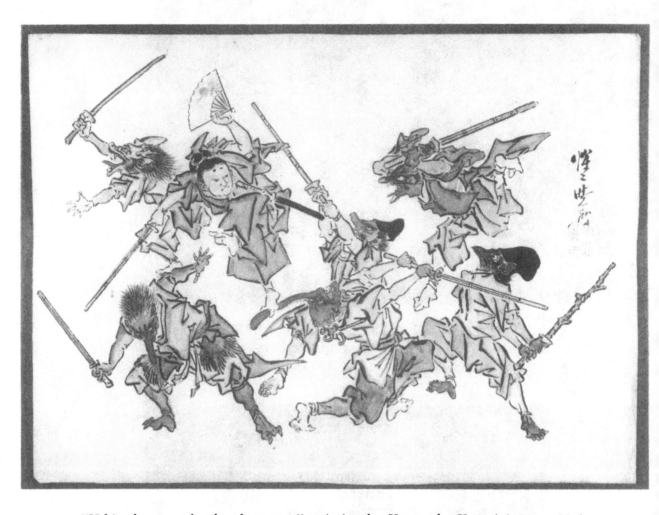

"Ushiwaka-maru battles the *tengu*," painting by Kawanabe Kyōsai (1831–1889).
The stance Ushiwaka-maru strikes with his sword is part of the *aiki-ken* repertoire. I
was taught this movement by Shirata Sensei, one of the disciples who accompanied
Morihei on his training sessions on Mount Kurama.

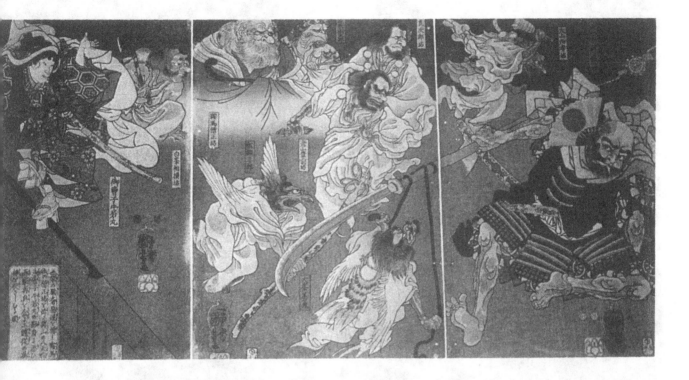

"Ushiwaka-maru thrashing the warrior monk Benkei on Kyoto's Gojō Bridge," woodblock print by Utagawa Kuniyoshi. Ushiwaka-maru, with the aid of an invisible (to Benkei) band of *tengu,* defeats the bandit-monk. After subjugating Benkei, Ushiwaka-maru made the monk his retainer. Morihei learned from Benkei as well as from Ushiwaka-maru's *tengu.* Once a teacher of Japanese classical dance called on Morihei and requested instruction in the art of *naginata.* Morihei had never really studied that weapon, but he agreed anyway, making an appointment with the teacher the following week. Morihei secluded himself in his room with a copy of "The Tale of Ushiwaka-maru and Benkei." Benkei's weapon of choice was the *naginata,* and he had never tasted defeat until his encounter with Ushiwaka-maru. Conjuring up Benkei's many battles in his mind, Morihei spent the day absorbing all of Benkei's techniques. Later he taught the dance teacher with confidence. When the dance teacher performed the *naginata* moves she had learned from Morihei, she received the highest praise from the audience for her marvelous skill.

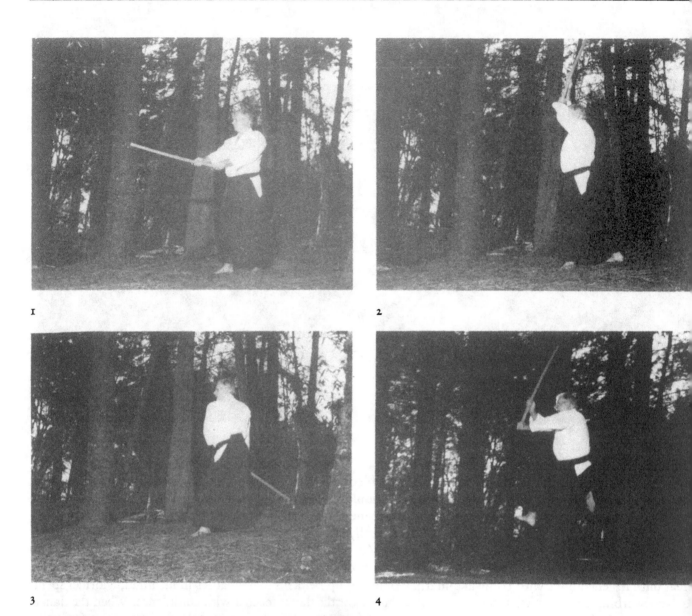

1

2

3

4

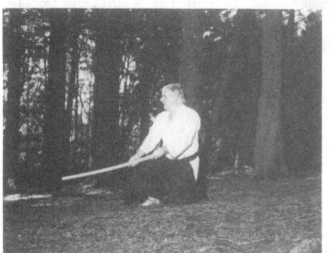

5

Tengu-tobigiri, "Flying Tengu Cut," taught to Ush
waka-maru by Shōjō-bo. A version of *tengu-tobigi*
is also used by *yamabushi* in rites of exorcism.

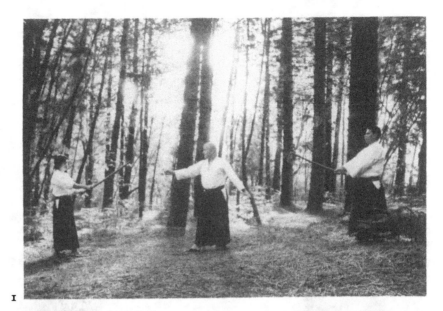

1

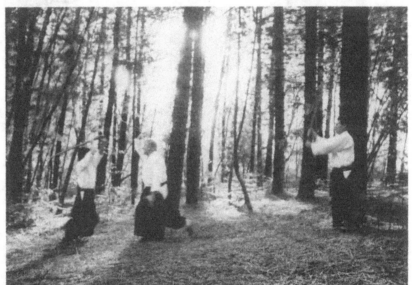

2

kidō is meant to be practiced out-
le as much as possible, in the forest
well as by the sea. Who knows?—a
gu may turn up.

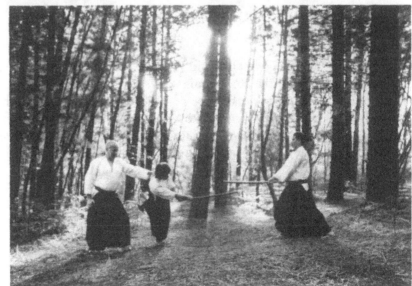

3

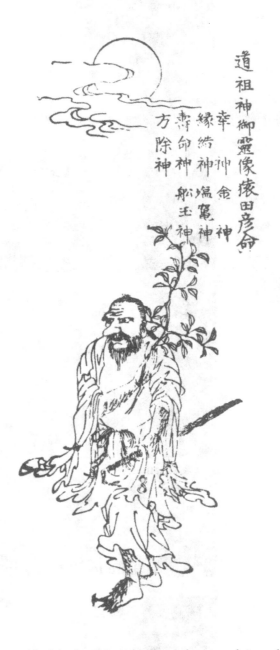

Morihei was also paid visits by Saruta-hiko-mikoto, a deity who may be considered the patron saint of *tengu*. Saruta-hiko points seekers in the right direction and otherwise assists religious wayfarers in their quest. On December 14, 1940, Saruta-hiko appeared to Morihei and announced that the Dragon King Ame-no-murakumo-kuki-samuhara Ryū-ō was going to take possession of Morihei's being.

RYŪ-Ō
THE DRAGON KING

*T*ENGU ARE PRETTY MUCH CONFINED TO JAPAN, BUT DRAGONS
and magic serpents thrive in all lands. Dragons are frightful creatures,
though, and in the West they have never been appreciated as being much more
than revolting beasts that beguile human beings and feast on damsels. In the
East, however, they were transformed into magnificent *nāgarāja,* "Dragon
Kings." The female counterpart is *nāgakanyā,* "Dragon Queen."

Nāga embody the life energy of the universe; they possess immense pent-
up power, which when released can be either tremendously productive, as
fertilizing rain and rich black earth, or terribly destructive, as typhoons and
raging waters. *Nāgarāja* (*nāgakanyā*) are forceful kings (queens) who jeal-
ously guard life's most precious treasures, bestowing the jewel of enlightenment only to the most worthy.

Morihei identified completely with his guardian Dragon King Ame-no-
murakumo-kuki-samuhara Ryū-ō.

> *Ame-no-murakumo* means literally "billowing clouds of heaven." Al-
> legorically, this phrase stands for the "mind-stuff" of the cosmos—
> a vast, scintillating intelligence that flows through and around us.
> In modern parlance, it is "the supreme consciousness."

> *Kuki* means "nine fierce spirits," code for the different levels of raw
> and subtle energy that fuel and propel the world.

Samuhara, literally "cold plain," actually means "awakened being." *Samu* is a reference to the crystal clarity of very cold air, in which everything stands out in sharp relief; *hara* is the "belly" of our own body and, simultaneously, that of the universe.

Ryū-ō, the Dragon King, is an *avatār,* "a deity who descends to earth" in times of great need. This kind of *avatār* manifests the truth in a flesh-and-blood fashion, something that we can see, hear, and touch as a true object. It further symbolizes one who can freely roam in all dimensions.

Once again we are dealing with both a grand vision and an actual presence. As explained above, Ame-no-murakumo-kuki-samuhara Ryū-ō incorporates the very truth of the universe, but it also appeared to us in the guise of a white-haired sage who imparted tangible treasures to his disciples in the way of techniques and oral instruction. Even though no longer physically present, Ame-no-murakumo-kuki-samuhara Ryū-ō continues to watch over us as the guardian angel of Aikidō.

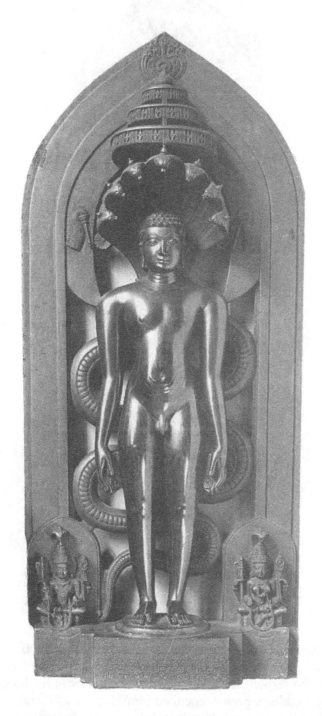

A Jain saint guarded by a *nāga*. Once converted to the *dharma*, the *nāga* become faithful protectors. The confident saint, his nakedness proclaiming his liberation from all attachment, assumes the posture of *kāyotsarga*, "setting free." In Japanese *budō*, this is called *shizen-tai*, "a totally natural stance." Prior to carving such a statue, the Indian artist would first bathe. After concentrating his mind, he would contemplate the slab and then mark its center. It is from this center, the *bindu*, that the image will arise and take shape as an auspicious whole.

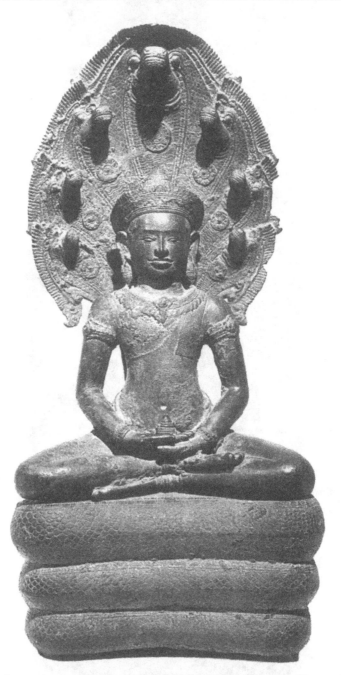

After attaining great enlightenment, Buddha abided in the bliss of *nirvāṇa* for a number of weeks. As he sat in repose under a banyan tree, a dreadful storm arose. The serpent king Muchalinda, stirred from his hole at the base of the tree by Buddha's presence, coiled himself around Gotama and spread out his prodigious hood to shelter the Awakened One from the wind and rain. Muchalinda's impenetrable armor shielded Buddha for the entire week the storm raged. When it finally abated, Muchalinda uncoiled himself and thereafter acted as Buddha's guardian. The *nāga* symbolizes the raw energy of nature that Buddha, through the authority of his enlightenment, was able to channel and direct. Buddha designated the *nāgarāja* as "guardians of the gate," and he entrusted them with the *Prajñāpāramitā* texts and magic *mantras*, to be revealed only to those ready for such potent transcendental wisdom.

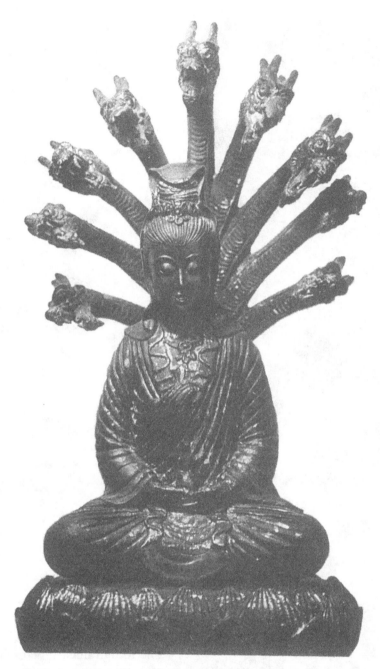

While *nāga* were portrayed as cobras in India, they were seen as dragons in China. Here a nine-headed Serpent King protects Kuan-yin, the Goddess of Compassion. As in the case of Muchalinda and the Buddha, here we have the most dynamic energy spiraling around the calmest center.

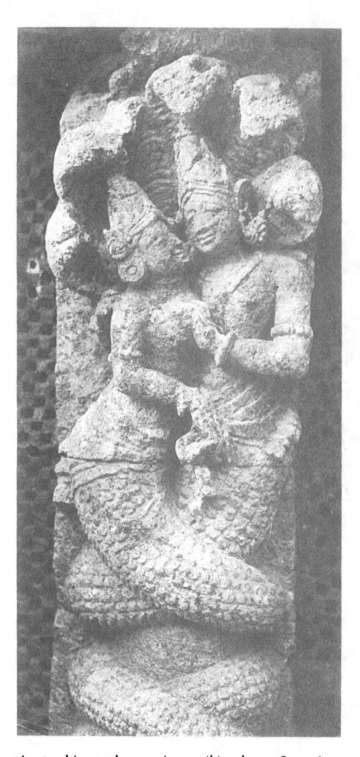

A *nāga* king and queen in an *aiki* embrace. Inextricably bound as one, the joyous couple represent the coming together of matter and spirit, the source of good health, fertility, and true enlightenment.

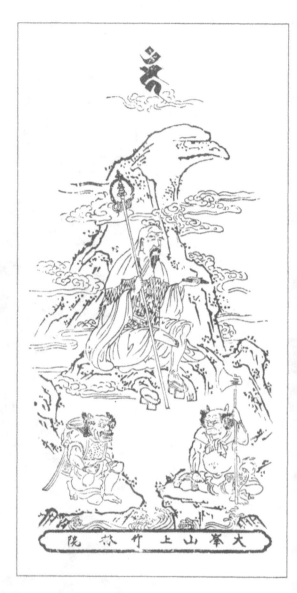

En-no-gyōja (c. 600 CE) the first *yamabushi*, wi his two demon attendants and sacred staff. The Si dham letter is HĀM, seed-syllable of Fudō Myō-The Indian master Nāgārjuna, who had been ini ated into the secrets of esoteric Buddhism by t *nāgarāja*, appeared in a vision to En-no-gyōja ar presented the Japanese hermit with the jewel of e lightenment. En-no-gyōja became a great and pov erful wizard: when highwaymen attacked him, I was able to shatter their swords and spears with h magic power. Morihei trained at many of the plac associated with this *yamabushi* master and studie En-no-gyōja's teachings. Morihei's guardian *nāg rāja* bestowed on him the secrets of *kototam* knowledge of all sounds.

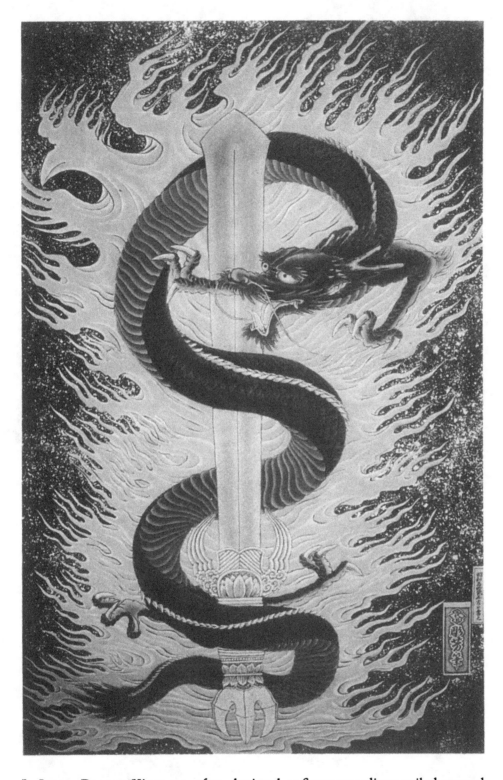

In Japan, Dragon Kings are often depicted as fierce guardians coiled around
the serene sword of wisdom. This is one way of representing Serpent Power
(*kuṇḍalinī*) ascending through the body. Painting by contemporary tattoo
master artist T. Kuronuma.

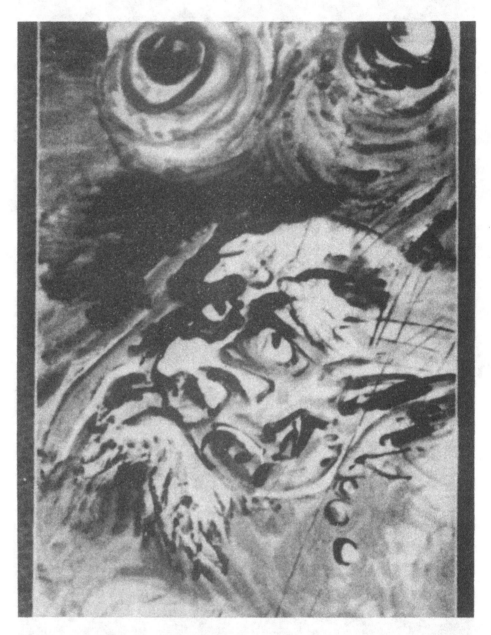

Morihei transfigured as Ame-no-murakumo-kuki-samuhara Ryū-ō, painted by Joyō Nozawa (1866–1937). This Dragon King is always present wherever Aikidō is sincerely practiced.

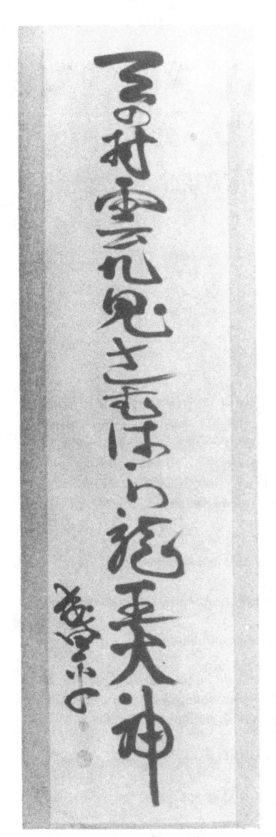

The Guardian Angel of Aikidō is presented in calligraphic form by Morihei: *Ame-no-murakumo-kuki-samuhara Ryū-ō Ō-Kami.*

MASAKATSU AGATSU KATSUHAYABI
TRUE VICTORY

*M*ASAKATSU AGATSU KATSUHAYABI IS THE MOTTO OF AIKIDŌ. *Masa* means "true, correct, straight"; *katsu* is "victory, triumph, success." *A* is "oneself," so the first half of the phrase may be literally translated as "True victory is victory over oneself." (This notion is akin to the teaching in Islam that "the lesser *jihad* is against the infidels; the greater *jihad* is against oneself.") Other possible interpretations of *Masakatsu Agatsu* include:

"Unflinching courage coupled with unflagging effort."

"Subdue your lower nature and you will always emerge victorious."

"The truth will free you from fear and self-doubt."

Haya is "swift, quick, dynamic," while *bi* (*hi*) is "sun, day, light." A literal translation of *katsuhayabi* (alternatively pronounced *kachihayahi*) would be "Day (Time) of Swift Victory!" This phrase additionally signifies:

"Accomplishment of many aims all at once."

"A state of being that transcends time and space."

"Each moment and every movement, vital and bright!"

Ultimately, everyone following the Path of Aiki must come up with his or her own understanding of this motto. Here are two *dōka* by Morihei on *Masakatsu Agatsu Katsuhayabi:*

> True Victory is Self Victory!
> Harmonize yourself with
> the heart of things
> and find salvation right
> inside your own body and soul!
>
> ———
>
> Contemplating this world
> I sometimes sigh with lament
> but then I continue my battle
> bathed in swirling light
> bringing closer the Day of Swift Victory!

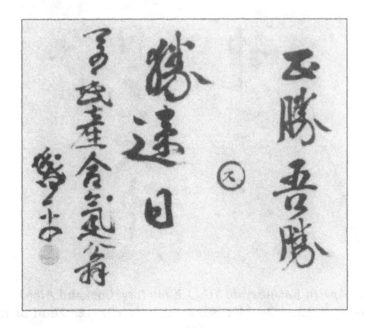

The *kototama* SU enveloped by *Masakatsu Agatsu* (right side) and *Katsuhayabi* (left side). If one is centered at the very heart of creation, surely he or she will emerge triumphant in any endeavor; one needs to realize this truth right here, right now. The calligraphy is signed "Morihei, the old fellow of Takemusu Aiki."

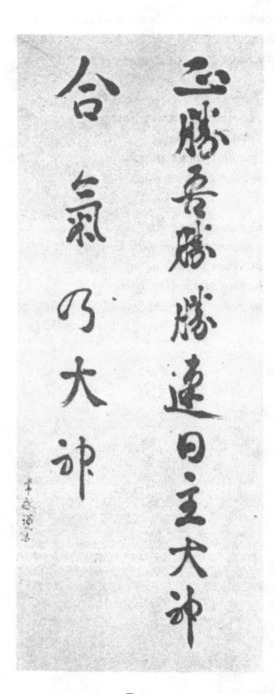

Masakatsu Agatsu Katsuhayabi SU Ō-Kami (first line) and *Aiki-no-Ō-Kami*
(second line), brushed by Morihei, a different representation of the same
principle.

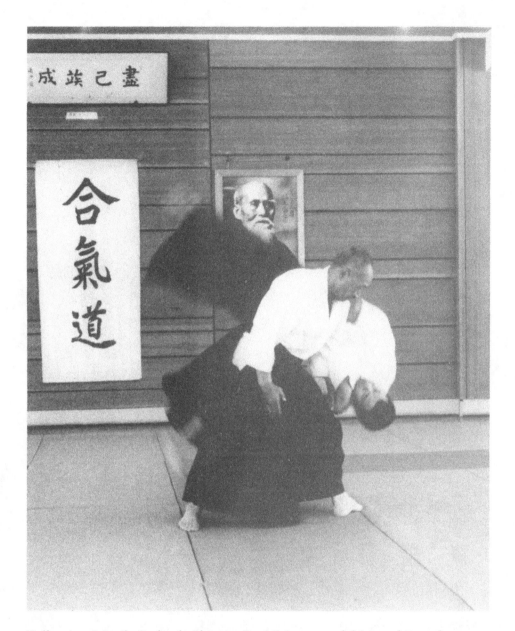

Following Morihei's lead, Shirata Sensei instructed his students always to maintain a state of *Masakatsu Agatsu* when executing the techniques: "If one's body and mind are true, the technique will be effective." Shirata Sensei once told us this tale: A young warrior visited a *yamabushi* who was rumored to possess the "Sword of Invincibility." The warrior begged the *yamabushi* to reveal the secret of the sword, and the wizard agreed, but only under the following conditions: "You must lead a chaste and frugal life, meditate for several hours each day, recite the special chants I give you, and train in the techniques I show you. Do this for twenty years, and I will reveal the secret of the sword." The intent warrior faithfully fulfilled his pledge and returned twenty years later. As promised, the wizard produced the magic sword. The warrior took it in his hands, held it a few minutes, and then gave it back—he no longer needed to rely on such a weapon.

WALKING THE PATH

THE PRACTICE OF AIKIDŌ

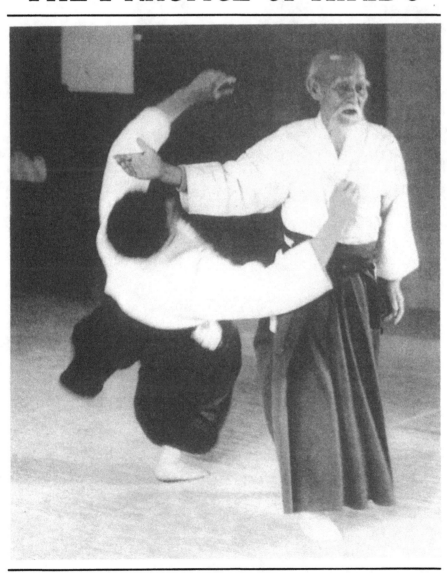

SHUGYŌ
CONSTANT TRAINING

THERE ARE NO SECRET TECHNIQUES IN AIKIDŌ. THE MANIFEST forms of Aikidō techniques are similar to those found in many other martial arts in different parts of the world. In the Uffizi Gallery, for instance, there is a famous statue depicting Greek wrestlers from the third century BCE, with one of them applying what Aikidō students call *sankyō* on the other. Morihei himself said, "I studied over thirty different kinds of martial arts, but following a transforming experience in 1940, I forgot every technique I had learned." In other words, the techniques flowed directly from the center of Morihei's being and were no longer fixed forms or standard patterns.

Late in life, Morihei led a training session, and all he appeared to be teaching was *ikkyō,* the most basic of all pins, variations of which are found in almost every other martial art. However, each time he demonstrated the technique, Morihei said, "Here is a new one." Finally, a perplexed student asked Morihei, "Sensei, all those techniques look the same." Morihei thundered back, "When you can see the difference between each of them, then you will understand the secret of Aikidō!"

The key to the secrets of Aikidō lies within—if your heart is true, your techniques will be true—but in order to mine those treasures we need a suitable path to follow, proper vehicles for training, and good teachers to point us in the right direction. For that we have, first of all, *keiko,* "the use of traditional wisdom to illuminate our present practice." Aikidō *keiko* has its own brand of distinctive exercises, which have been outlined in dozens of technical manuals, so there is no need to discuss the details here. The attitude one has toward *keiko* is more important than the contents of the training, and Morihei often spoke of the four virtues of *keiko:* bravery, wisdom, love, and empathy.

Bravery is first, for we need to be strong and determined enough to make a firm commitment to practice. We need sufficient valor to help us contend with, and overcome, the myriad obstacles that block our path. Wisdom is acquired through meditation and wide-ranging study; wisdom enables us to make intelligent decisions and to maintain things in proper perspective. When one's practice is sound and balanced, a natural kind of love forms between our teacher and our fellow trainees. We also fall in love with our Way, and become completely devoted to it. At the highest levels of training, a profound empathy is felt for all creatures, along with the fervent hope that everyone else, too, will follow the Way to the end. As mentioned previously, one of the meanings of Aikidō is, "Arm in arm, let's travel the Path together"—like a bodhisattva we want all others to reach the goal with us.

Morihei spoke of *keiko* not as a harsh regimen and an ascetic ordeal but as *misogi,* a means to restore our link to the universe. Morihei further emphasized that *keiko* is a matter of faith and trust, helping us realize our incredible potential and to experience the joy of being. Morihei likened *keiko* to standing on the "Floating Bridge of Heaven" that links the inner and outer worlds; there we must emulate Izanagi and Izanami and create fresh techniques of harmony. In good *keiko,* tension is removed, the balance between fire and water is restored, and pleasure is experienced.

Sometimes a more concentrated effort is needed in our practice. Morihei wrote, "Iron is full of impurities that weaken it: through forging, it becomes steel and is transmuted into a razor-sharp blade. Human beings develop in the same fashion." Such forging, *tanren,* can take a variety of forms, most typically as a special daily practice (such as 1,000 cuts of the sword) or an intensive retreat (like the ones Morihei made on Mount Kurama).

It is also essential to incorporate four qualities into one's *keiko.* The diamond quality is hard, precise, stable. Beginners should rely mostly on diamond techniques in order to build a solid base. (*Adamas,* the Greek word for diamond, also means "invincible.") The willow quality is more flexible, the principle that lies at the heart of Judō. The flowing quality is dynamic and more free-form than the first two, like water flowing in a valley stream smoothly between the rocks. The *ki* quality is "empty," a power so subtle and refined (on the highest level) that it is hardly necessary to touch one's partner at all. It is interesting to apply the four qualities individually to the same technique, but this is something that cannot be adequately illustrated in a book. Such things belong in the realm of *kuden,* "secret oral instruction."

The real meaning of *kuden* is person-to-person, heart-to-heart transmission. One has to experience the texture of the teaching—touch it, grasp it, feel it in the bones. The finest instructors teach by example—"What you are is far more important than what you say"—and there is no substitute for intimate, face-to-face contact with the art.

Life-long walking of the Path is called *shugyō* in Japanese. Morihei taught, "In your training, do not be in a hurry, for it takes a minimum of ten years to master the basics and advance to the first rung. Never think of yourself as an all-knowing perfected master; you must continue to train daily with your friends and students and progress together in the Way of Harmony."

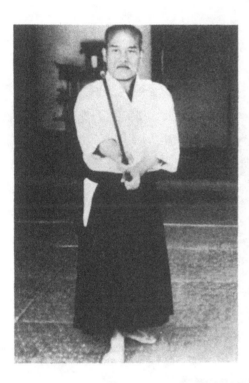 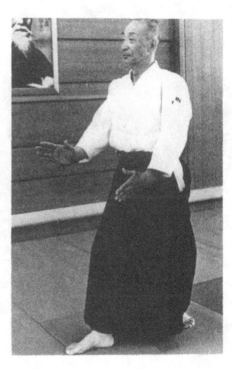

Left: "A good stance reflects a proper state of mind." The basic Aikidō stance is derived from the *hanmi kamae* of classical swordsmanship, demonstrated here by Morihei. In the old days, many a contest was decided as soon as the opponents assumed their respective stances—a weak stance immediately provided a skilled swordsman with an opening in which to strike. On the other hand, if one's opponent displayed no such weakness, it was best to withdraw and beat a hasty retreat. *Right:* The stance assumed in body techniques, demonstrated here by Shirata Sensei, should be equally strong and stable.

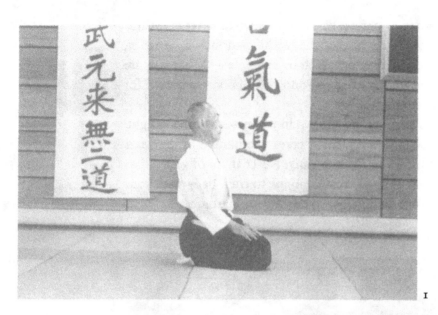

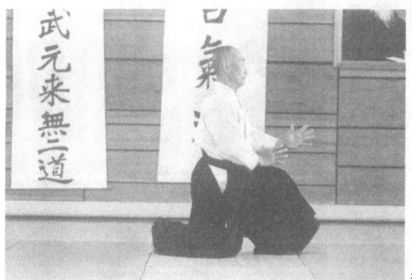

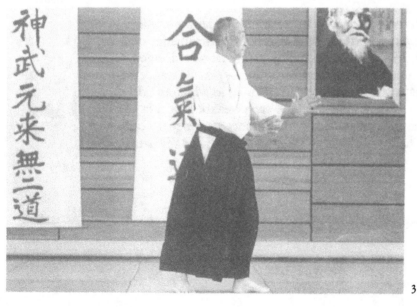

Sitting, rising, or standing, one should always maintain *fudō-shin*, "an imperturbable mind and an unbreakable posture."

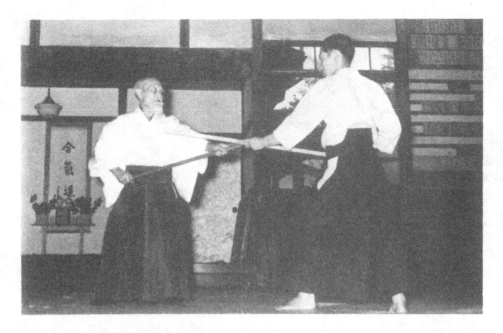

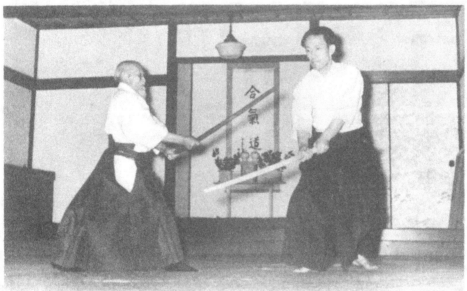

Morihei, practicing here with his son Kisshomaru, taught that training with the *jō* fostered good intuition (knowing when to enter), while training with the *ken* developed good resolution (knowing how to apply and complete the technique). The *jō* initiated the movement and the *ken* defined it.

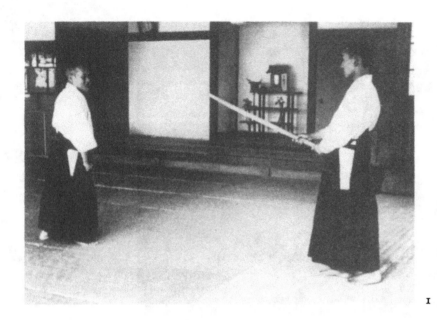

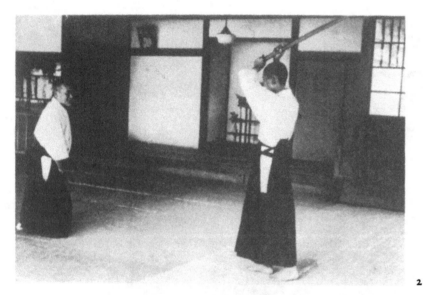

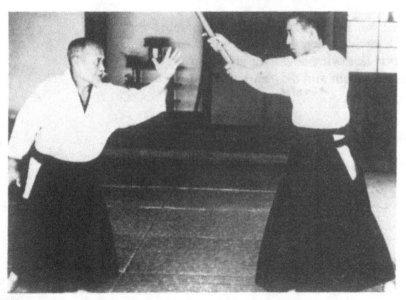

One of the secrets of Aikidō is the abilit
to lead one's partner. Morihei spoke o
"inviting your partner to strike" (1, 2
Once the opponent is committed, a tech
nique can be applied (3). The art o
"drawing out and leading" is difficult t
master, though, requiring years of soli
practice. For a beginning student in an
discipline, training is 90 percent tech
nique and 10 percent intuition; for
master the percentage is reversed—9
percent intuition and 10 percent tech
nique.

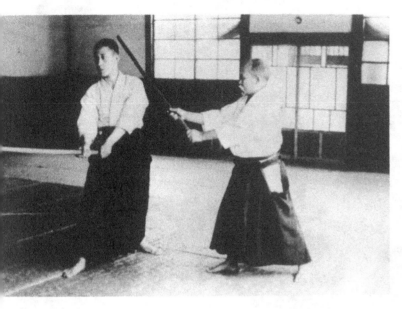

Morihei emphasized entering at just the right angle, literally and figuratively. A 90-degree entry against a head-on attack, as illustrated here by Morihei, is very effective. Such a movement brings one into the opponent's *shikaku*, "dead angle," from which no counterattack is possible. Aikidō is largely a matter of always being in the right place.

epending on who tells the story, Morihei is ported to have said that *atemi* was either percent, 60 percent, or 99 percent of an fective technique. Rather than a devastat-g blow, however, *atemi* should be thought as a neutralizing force, making it easier to ide the attack.

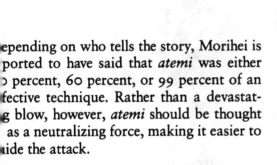

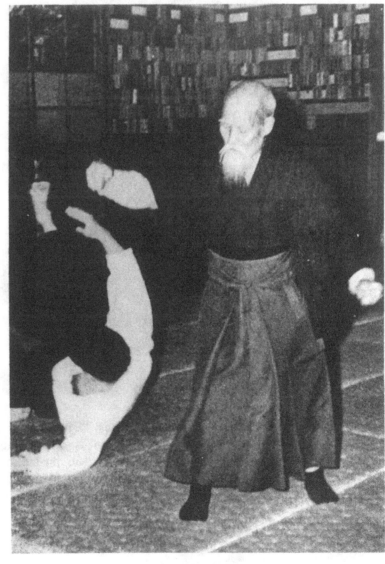

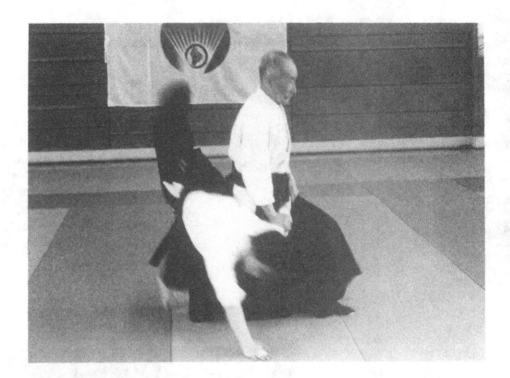

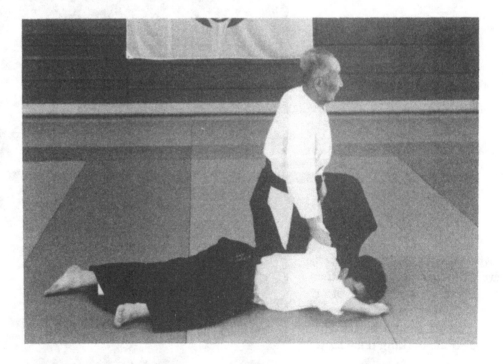

Shirata Sensei used to tell us, "Throw your partner without throwing, pin him without pinning—rely on *Masakatsu Agatsu*." That is, if your mind is clear and your movements are true, the technique accomplishes itself—*Katsu Hayabi*. Here, Sensei's technique is true (effective), good (his partner is not injured), and beautiful (in perfect proportion).

THE SIX PILLARS

AIKIDŌ TECHNIQUES REVOLVE AROUND SIX BASIC PILLARS: *shihō-nage, irimi, kaiten, kokyū, osae-waza,* and *ushiro-waza.* These techniques represent the grammar of Aikidō, the language in which the tradition is formulated and expressed. These techniques are not set in stone, however; they are flexible and expansive reference points. Each pillar incorporates many different features, and shares some aspects with one or more of the other pillars. In a regular training session, it is advisable to include at least one technique from each of the pillars in order to maintain good *aiki* balance.

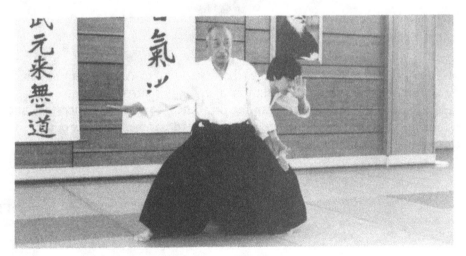

Shirata Sensei demonstrating a *kaiten* movement,
one of the six pillars of Aikidō.

SHIHŌ-NAGE: *GRATITUDE*

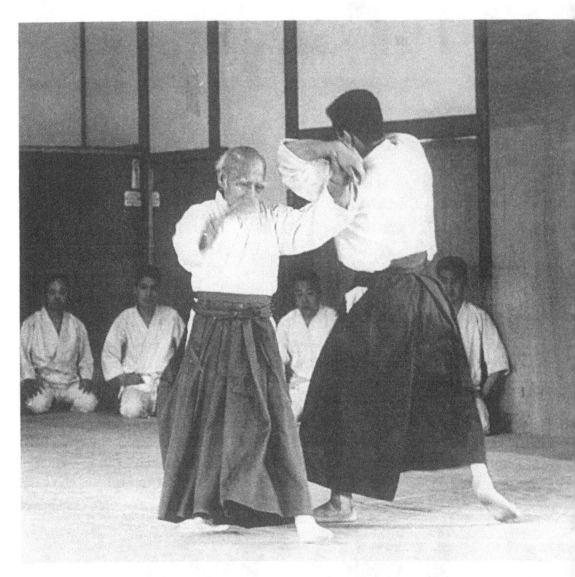

Morihei demonstrating *shihō-nage,* the first pillar of Aikidō techniques. *Shihō* means "four directions," symbolizing appreciation of the *kami* surrounding us, as well as the four gratitudes: toward the universe, the source of all life; toward our ancestors and parents, who are responsible for our individual existence; toward nature, which provides our daily sustenance; toward other human beings who help us survive in society.

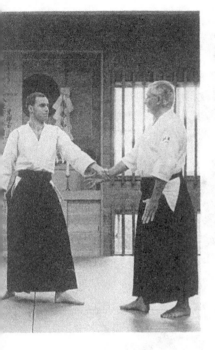

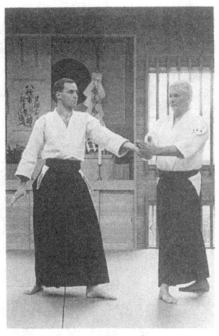
2

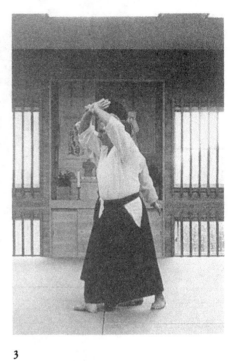
3

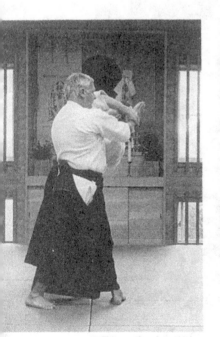

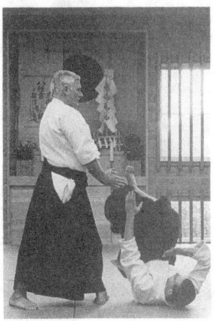
5

Shirata Sensei often described Aikidō as *inori no budō*, "the martial art of prayer," a prayer that generates light (wisdom) and heat (compassion). It is possible to perform *shihō-nage* as an act of worship.

IRIMI: *ENTERING*

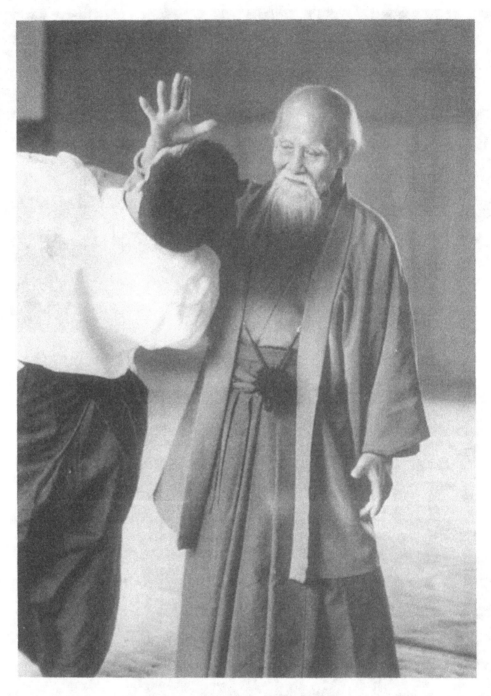

Irimi techniques constitute the second pillar of Aikidō. One has to enter deeply, physically and spiritually, against an attack, becoming one with the aggressive force and thereby diffusing it.

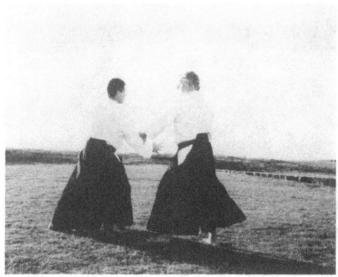

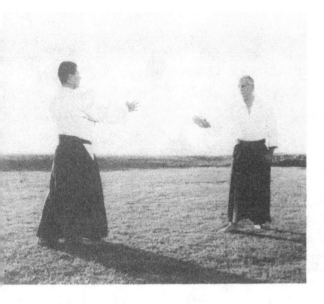

2

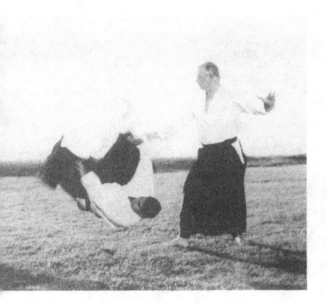

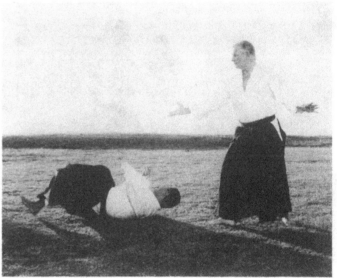

4

An example of a precise triangular *irimi* against a *shomen* attack.

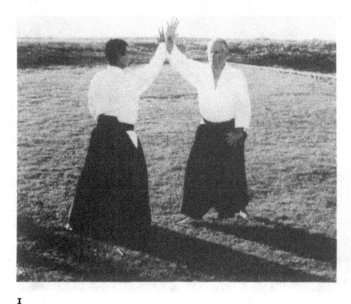

1

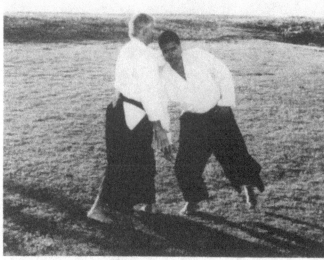

2

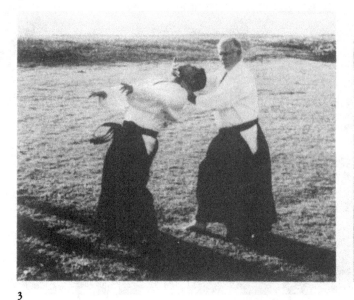

3

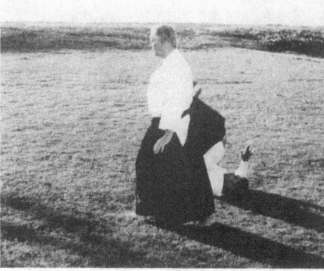

4

In circular *irimi* movements such as this, one rotates in a big spiral, naturally drawing one's partner in (2), around (3), and then down (4).

AITEN: *OPEN AND TURN*

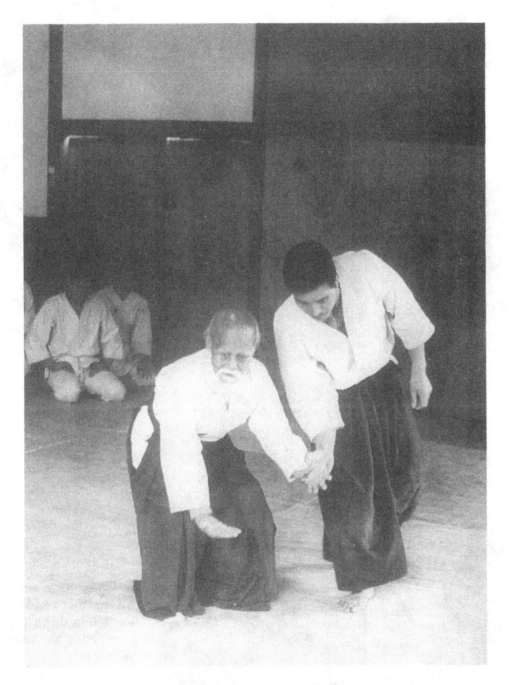

The third pillar of Aikidō is *kaiten* techniques. *Kai* means "open"—as in "opening a path around an aggressive force"—and *ten* is "turn"—as in "turn things around in your favor." Late in life, Morihei's *kaiten* movements often included a big dip, a wavelike motion that made the techniques even more effective.

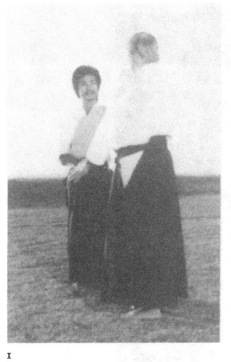

1

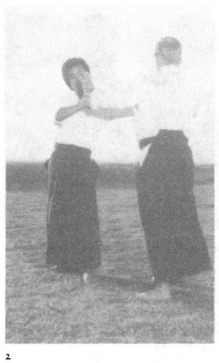

2

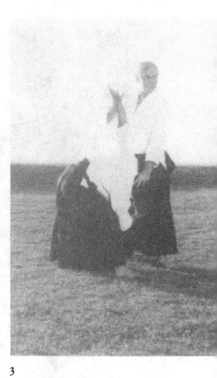

3

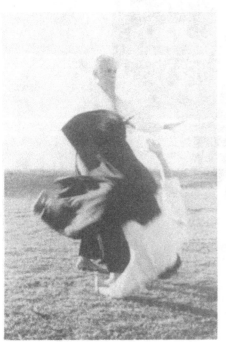

4

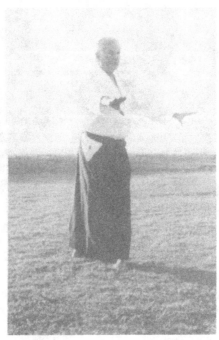

5

In *kaiten nage,* one first opens
his partner's side (2) and the
turns him down (3) and out (4
completing the technique in *za*
shin (5).

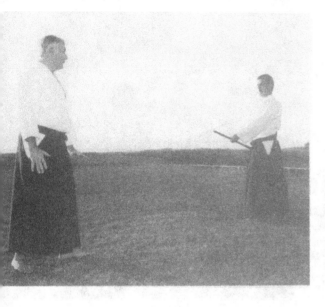

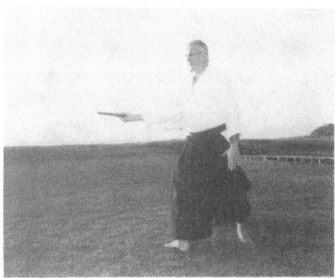

2

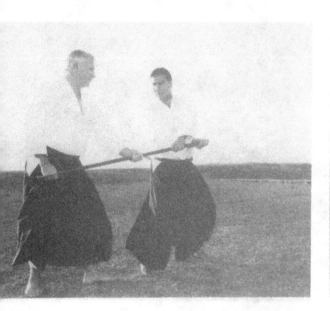

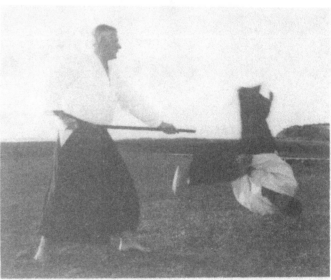

4

Here is a double *kaiten* turn against a *jō* attack (1). First to the outside (2) and then back to the inside (3).

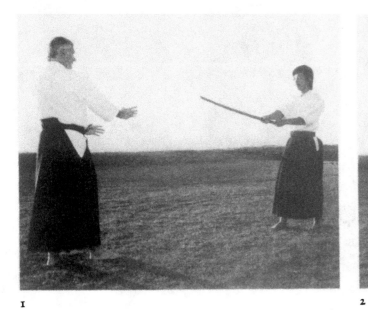

1

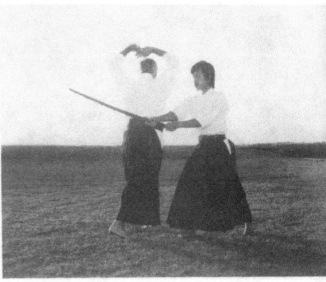

2

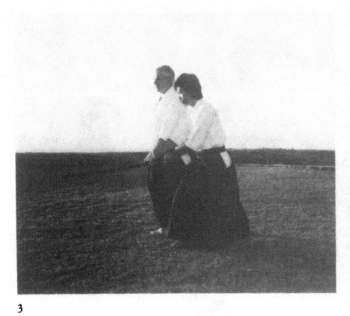

3

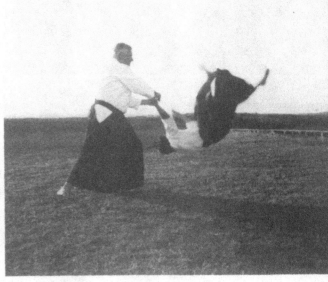

4

Against a sword attack (1), a two-step *irimi* move (2, 3) is combined with a *kaiten* throw (4).

OKYŪ: *BREATH POWER*

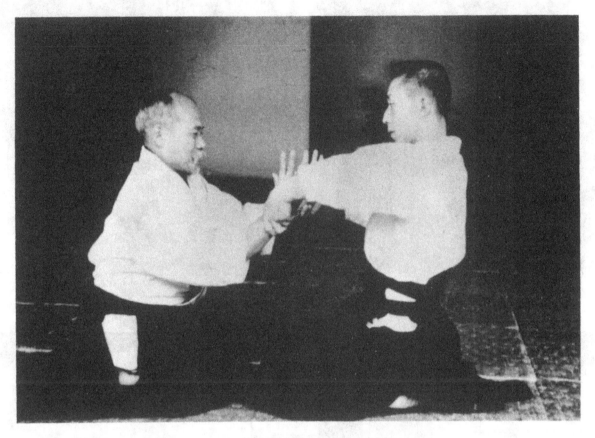

Kokyū techniques form the fourth pillar of Aikidō.
Here, Morihei demonstrates *suwari kokyū-hō*.

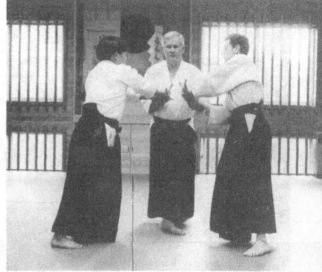

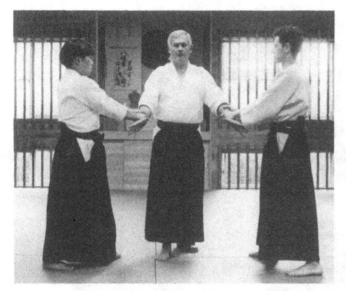

1

2

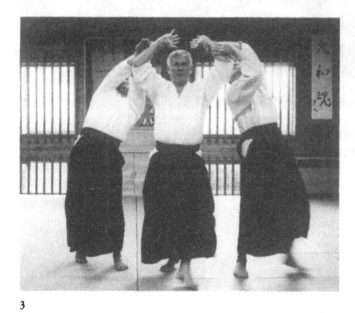

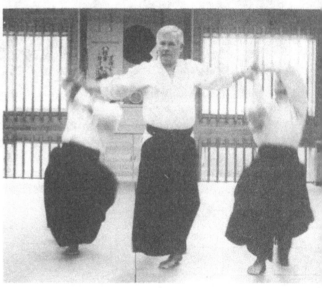

3

4

Standing *kokyū-hō* techniques practiced with two *uke* in two aspects, diamond (*above*) and willow (*opposite*).

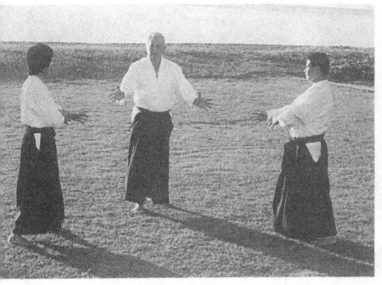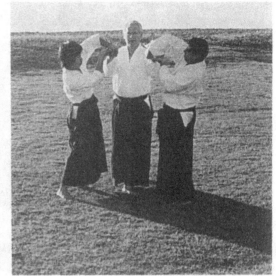

2

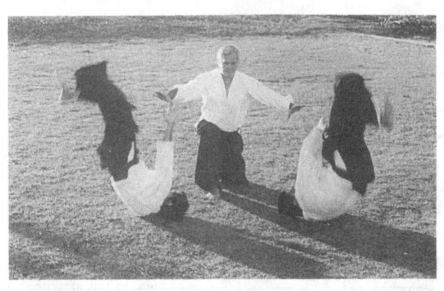

3

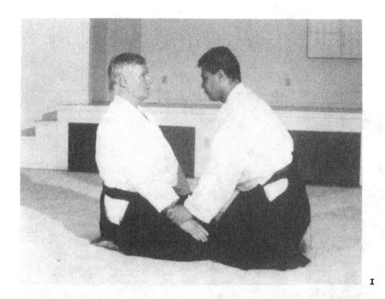

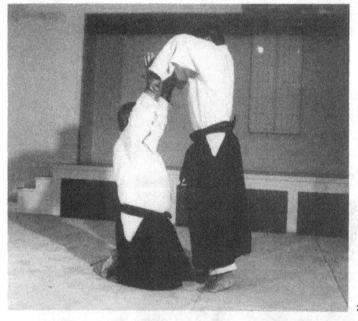

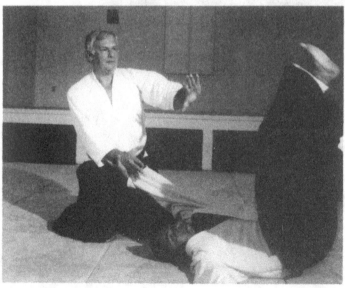

Kokyū power is best developed in *suwari kokyū-h* techniques. In this exercise, *tori* lets *uke* pin hi full force from above (1). *Tori* employs breat power to raise *uke* all the way up (2), and then *uk* can be thrown in any direction, in this case to th front (3).

SAE-WAZA: *FIRM CONTROL*

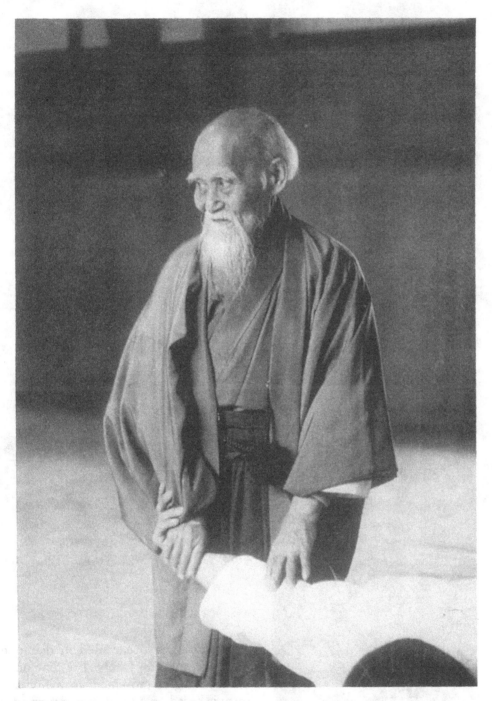

Osae-waza, "pinning techniques," make up the fifth pillar of Aikidō. Pins represent firm control. Morihei emphasized the health-promoting properties of the various pins: they stimulate the joints, stretch the muscles, and otherwise invigorate the limbs.

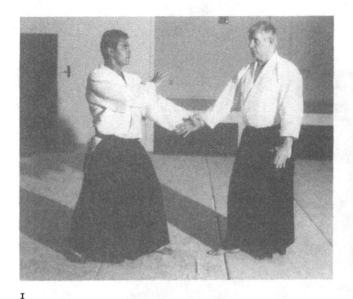

1

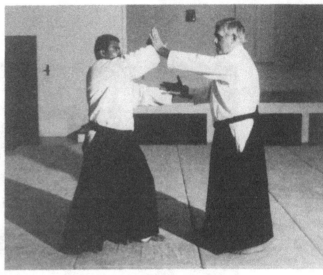

2

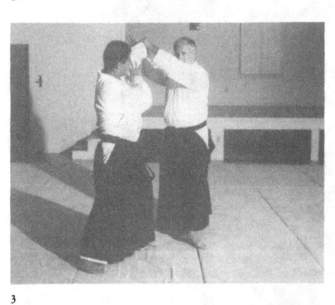

3

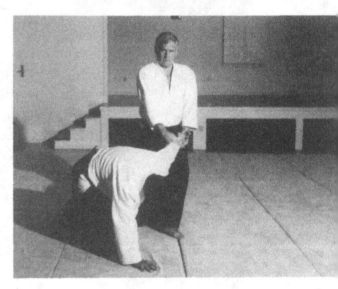

4

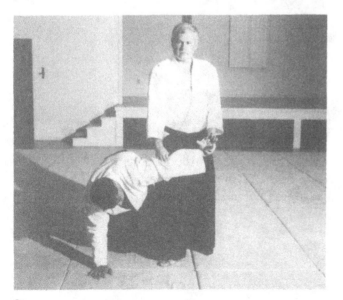

5

Katate-dori ikkyō executed in diamond (*above*) an flowing (*opposite*) forms. The diamond form is base on a 90-degree movement to the outside; the flowin form is based on a 90-degree movement to the inside.

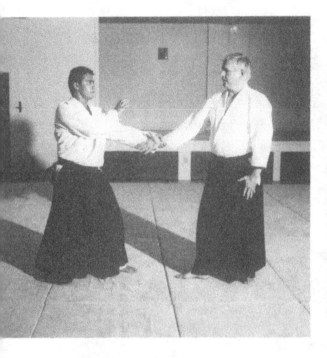

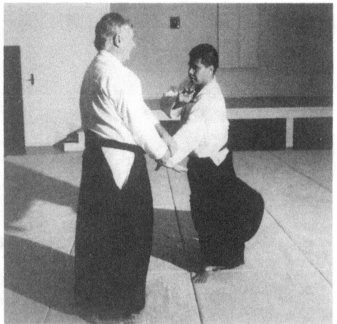

2

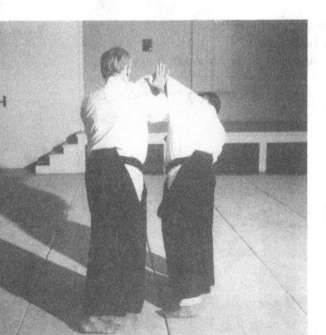

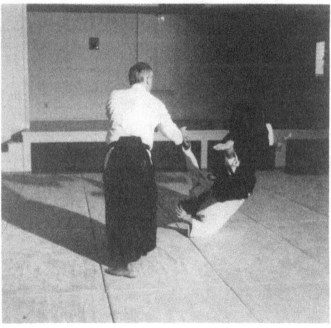

4

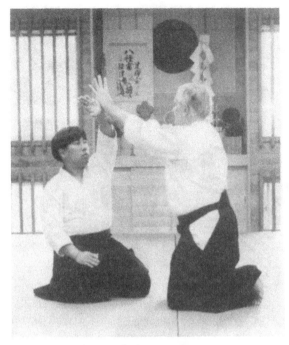

1

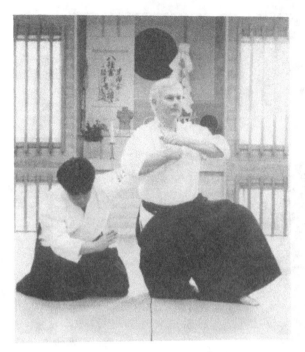

2

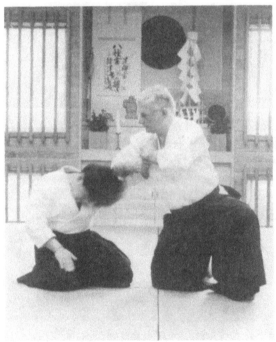

3

One meaning of *mudrā*, the hand gestures used in Tantra, is "lock," and here we have the Aikidō *nikkyō mudrā*. Although it appears to be a linear movement, actually *nikkyō* is applied in a spiral motion as if "embracing the earth."

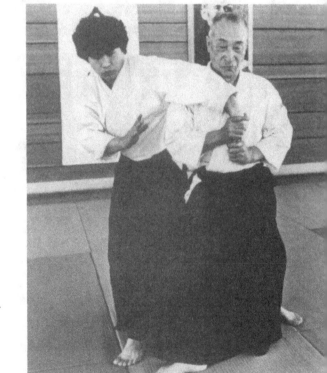

Shirata Sensei and his *sankyō mudrā*, exemplifying perfect control, correct form, and unity of body and mind.

SHIRO-WAZA: *SIXTH SENSE*

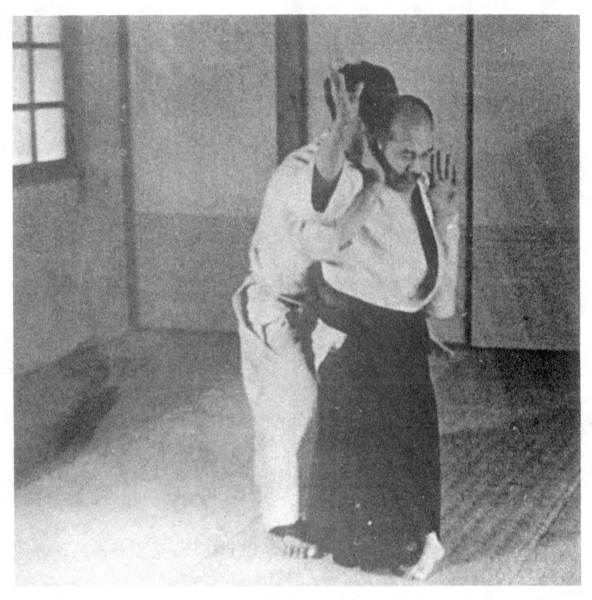

Ushiro-waza, the sixth pillar of Aikidō, foster the development of one's sixth sense.

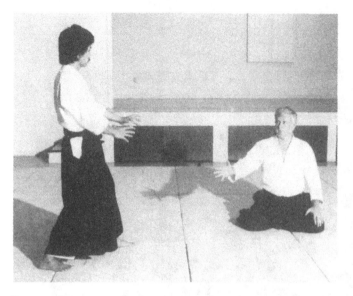

1

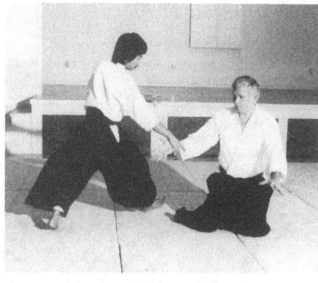

2

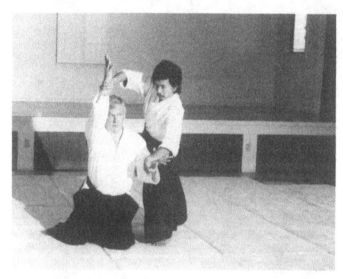

3

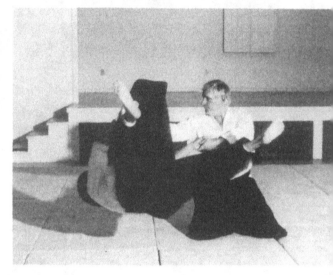

4

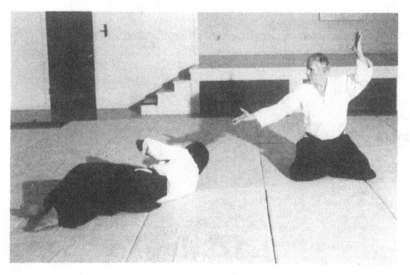

5

Ushiro ryōte-dori kokyū nage executed in *hanmi-hantachi*. Morihei considered the practice of the techniques in a seated position to be very important. In the old days he told his students, "When I cannot lead the practice, confine yourselves to seated techniques. It will make your legs stronger and you have to learn how to move just right to make the techniques work."

KIAI: *THE INTEGRATED SYSTEM*

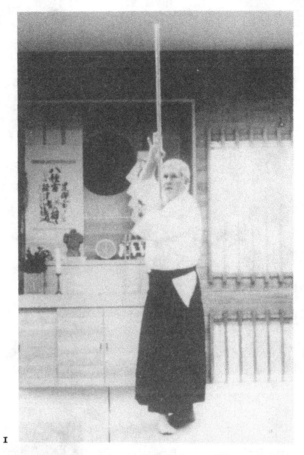

1

iai means "integrated principles." The movements of *aiki-ken, aiki-jō,* and *taijutsu* should be integrated and interchangeable. The *hassō* stance (1) has many applications in the body techniques (2).

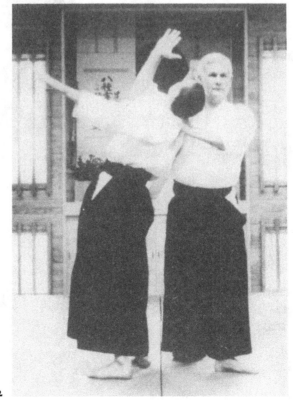

2

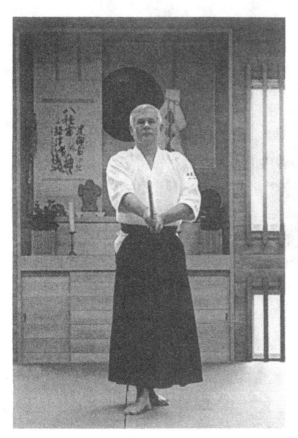

1

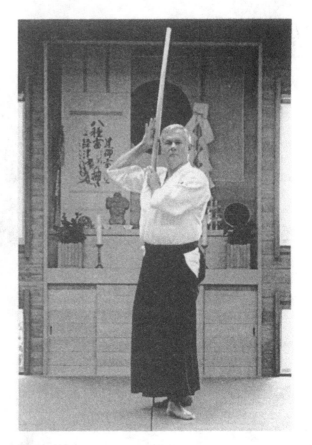

2

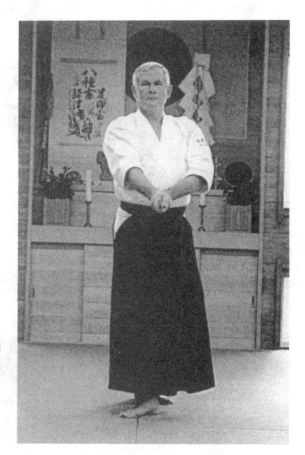

3

From a *seigan* stance (1), step back and assume the *hassō* posture (2), and then step forward with a powerful strike (3).

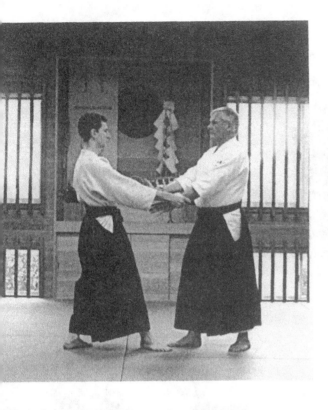

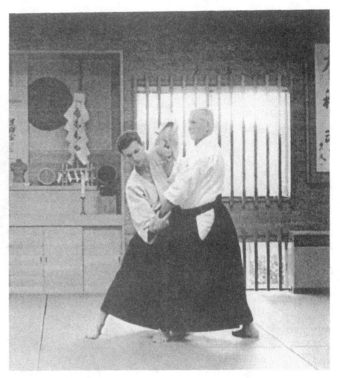

2

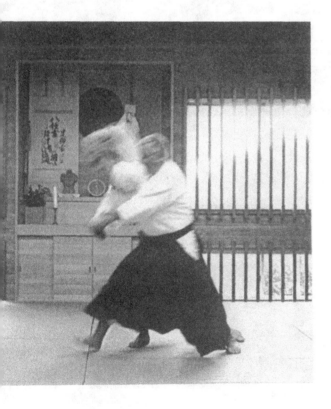

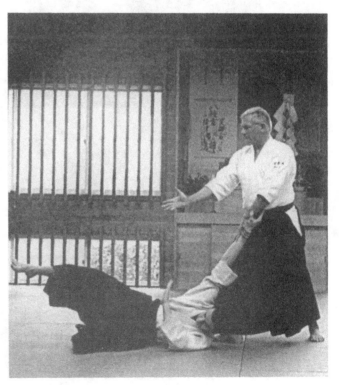

4

The same movement applied to a body technique, *ryōte-dori* (1). Step back and assume a *hassō* posture (2), then step forward (3) and throw (4).

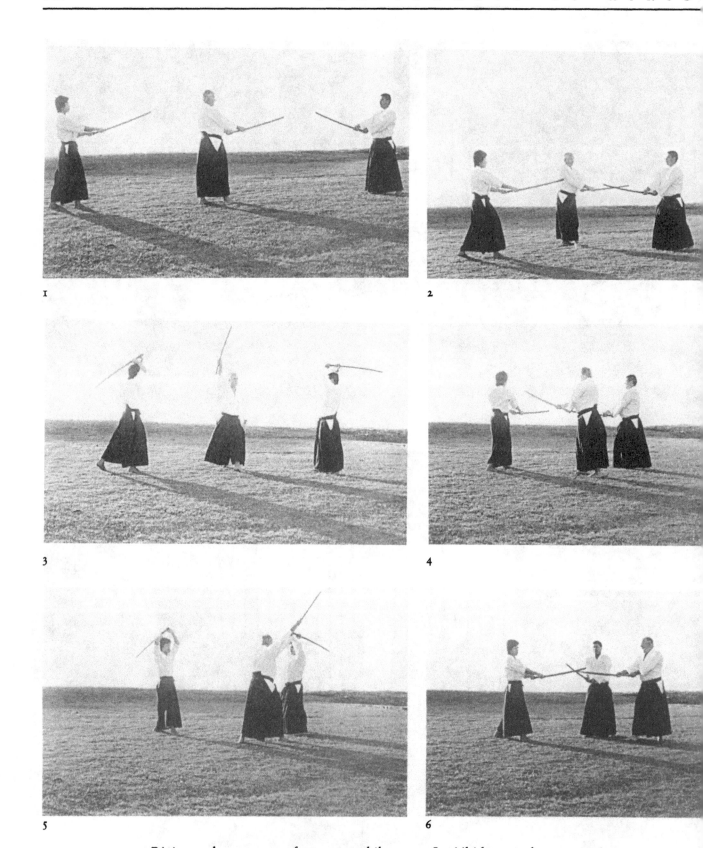

Riai sword movements for *omote shihō-nage*. In Aikidō, we always remain aware of attackers front and back, right and left.

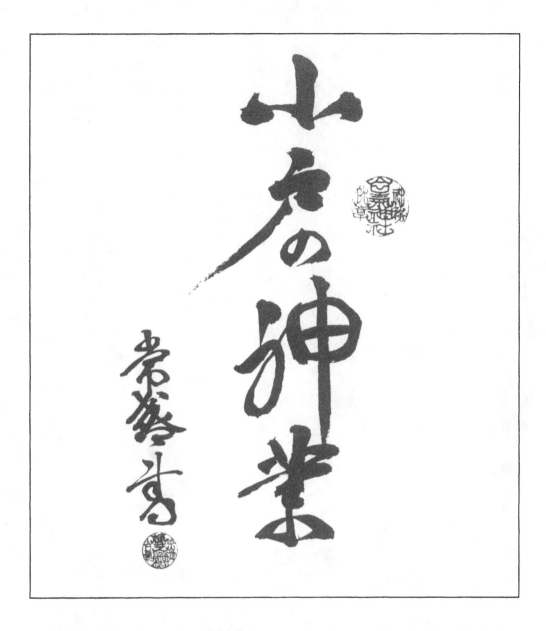

Odo-no-Kamuwaza, the "Divine Techniques of ODO," brushed by Morihei. One of the meanings of ODO is being in just the right place, physically and spiritually; in that state, techniques can really seem miraculous.

APPENDIXES

KOTOTAMA

The Secret Sounds of Aikidō

Based on the teachings of Morihei, I have formulated these methods of *kototama* chanting for use in regular Aikidō training.[1]

Following the lead of the instructor, the members of the *dōjō* chant in unison the *kototama*[2]

SU-U-U-U-U-YU-MU.

Then the *kototama*

A-O-U-E-I

are pronounced slowly and strongly three times. This is followed by the *kototama*[3]

MA-SA-KA-TSU
A-GA-TSU
KA-TSU-HA-YA-BI

---

1. *Kototama: The Secret Sounds of Aikidō*, a cassette recording of these chants, is available from *Aikidō Today Magazine*. See Suggested Reading.
2. Refer to pages 17–19, 24. Japanese vowels are pronounced as follows: *A* as in "ah," *O* as in "rose," *U* as in "true," *E* as in "grey," and *I* as in "machine."
3. Refer to pages 104–106.

which are voiced separately, strongly and slowly, one time apiece. The concluding *kototama*[4] is:

A-I-KI-O-O-KA-MI.

This concludes the abbreviated version of the chanting. In the longer version, the *kototama*

MA-SA-KA-TSU A-GA-TSU KA-TSU-HA-YA-BI

is employed, rhythmically chanted thirteen times. This is followed by the A-UN *kototama,* voiced as OM, and repeated three, twenty-five, or fifty times.[5] Next is the *kototama*[6]

NA-MU A-ME-NO-MU-RA-KU-MO
KU-KI SA-MU-HA-RA RYU-U-O-O

chanted thirteen times. This sequence ends with the *kototama*

A-I-KI-O-O-KA-MI

Another *kototama* practice employed by Morihei and sometimes adopted in Aikidō *dōjō* is the series:

HI-FU-MI-YO-I-MU-NA-YA-KO-TO-MO-CHI-RO

(also voiced as)

HITO-FUTA-MI-YO-ITSU-MUYU-NANA-
YAA-KOKONO-TARI-MOMO-CHI-YOROZU

literally:

1-2-3-4-5-6-7-
8-9-10-100-1,000-10,000

This was the chant sung by Ame-no-Umezu while she was dancing on the drum.[7] It has a variety of interpretations, ranging from the erotic—"See, all you gods, my divine splendor: behold my bosom and thighs"—to the mysti-

4. Refer to page 35.
5. Refer to pages 47–49.
6. Refer to pages 95–96.
7. Refer to page 23.

cal—One (Spirit), Two (Heat and Light), Three (Materialization), Four (World), Five (Becoming), Six (Fermenting), Seven (Earth), Eight (Ascending), Nine (Heaven), Ten (Complete Cycle), One Hundred (Eternal Mother), One Thousand (Eternal Father), Ten Thousand (The Continual Birth of Myriad Existence). Like most *mantra,* this *kototama* is best left unexplained, for the meaning will gradually reveal itself to the practitioner.

From his studies of Shingon Buddhism, Morihei learned to chant the *Hannya Shingyō,* one of the most potent Buddhist *kototama:*

MA-KA HAN-NYA HA-RA-MI-TA SHIN-GYŌ
KAN-JI-ZAI BO-SA-TSU GYŌ JIN HAN-NYA HA-
RA-MI-TA JI SHŌ KEN GO-ON KAI KŪ DO IS-SAI
KU YA-KU SHA-RI-SHI SHI-KI FU I KŪ KŪ FU I
SHI-KI SHI-KI SO-KU ZE KŪ KŪ SO-KU ZE SHI-
KI JU SŌ GYŌ SHI-KI YA-KU BU NYO ZE SHA-
RI-SHI ZE SHŌ-HŌ KŪ SŌ FU-SHŌ FU-ME-TSU
FU-KU FU-JŌ FU-ZŌ FU-GEN ZE KO KŪ CHŪ MU
SHI-KI MU JU SŌ GYŌ SHI-KI MU GEN NI BI
ZES-SHIN NI MU SHI-KI SHŌ KŌ MI SO-KU HŌ
MU GEN KAI NAI SHI MU I SHI-KI KAI MU MU-
MYŌ YA-KU MU MU-MYŌ JIN NAI SHI MU RŌ
SHI YA-KU MU RŌ SHI JIN MU KU SHŪ ME-TSU
DŌ MU CHI YA-KU MU TO-KU I MU SHO-TO-KU
KO BO-DAI-SAT-TA E HAN-NYA HA-RA-MI-TA
KO SHIN MU KEI-GE MU KEI-GE KO MU U KU-
FU ON-RI IS-SAI TEN-DŌ MU SŌ KU GYŌ NE-
HAN SAN-ZE SHŌ BU-TSU E HAN-NYA HA-RA-
MI-TA KO TO-KU A-NO-KU-TA-RA SAM-MYA-KU
SAM-BO-DAI KO CHI HAN-NYA HA-RA-MI-TA
ZE DAI JIN SHU ZE DAI MYŌ SHU ZE MU-JŌ
SHU ZE MU-TŌ-DŌ SHU NŌ JO IS-SAI KU SHIN-
JI-TSU FU KO KO SETSU HAN-NYA HA-RA-MI-TA
SHU SO-KU ZE-TSU SHU WA-TSU GYA-TEI GYA-
TEI HA-RA-GYA-TEI HA-RA-SO-GYATE BO-JI SO-
WA-KA HAN-NYA SHIN-GYŌ.

For those who wish to chant in English:

THE HEART SUTRA

THE BO-DHI-SATT-VA OF COM-PAS-SION, MOV-ING IN THE
DEEP-EST WIS-DOM, CLEAR-LY SAW THAT THE FIVE HEAPS ARE

EMPTY AND THUS PASSED OVER ALL SUF-FER-ING AND DIS-
TRESS. O SHA-RI-PU-TRA, FORM IS NOT DIF-FER-ENT FROM
EMP-TI-NESS, EMP-TI-NESS IS NOT DIF-FER-ENT FROM FORM.
FORM IS EMP-TI-NESS, EMP-TI-NESS IS FORM. FEEL-ING,
THOUGHT, VO-LI-TION, AND CON-SCIOUS-NESS ARE ALL LIKE
THIS. O SHA-RI-PU-TRA, ALL THINGS ARE EMP-TY: THEY HAVE
NO BIRTH, NO DEATH, NO TAINT, NO PUR-I-TY, NO IN-CREASE,
NO DE-CREASE. HENCE: IN EMP-TI-NESS THERE IS NO FORM,
NO FEEL-ING, NO THOUGHT, NO VO-LI-TION, NO CON-SCIOUS-
NESS; NO EYES, NO EARS, NO NOSE, NO TONGUE, NO BO-DY,
NO MIND; NO COL-OR, NO SOUNDS, NO SMELL, NO TASTE, NO
TOUCH, NO IN-TELL-ECT; NO REALM OF SIGHT RIGHT
THROUGH NO REALM OF CON-SCIOUS-NESS; NO IG-NOR-ANCE
AND NO EX-TINC-TION OF IG-NOR-ANCE; NO OLD AGE AND
DEATH AND NO EX-TINC-TION OF OLD AGE AND DEATH: NO
SUF-FER-ING, NO CRAV-ING, NO CEAS-ING, AND NO PATH; NO
WIS-DOM AND NO AT-TAIN-MENT. WITH NO-THING TO BE AT-
TAINED, BO-DHI-SATT-VAS RE-LY ON GREAT WIS-DOM WITH
MINDS FREE OF HIN-DRANCE. FREE OF HIN-DRANCE THERE IS
NO FEAR. FAR BE-YOND DE-LU-SIVE VIEWS THEY FIND NIR-VA-
NA. ALL BUD-DHAS OF THE THREE WORLDS RE-LY ON GREAT
WIS-DOM AND THUS OB-TAIN SU-PREME EN-LIGHT-EN-MENT.
THERE-FORE KNOW THAT THE GREAT WIS-DOM HERE IS THE
MOST DI-VINE MAN-TRA, THE BRIGHT-EST MAN-TRA, THE
HIGH-EST MAN-TRA, THE IN-COM-PAR-ABLE MAN-TRA THAT AL-
LAYS ALL SUF-FER-ING. THIS IS THE TRUTH, NOT FALSE-HOOD.
SO PRO-CLAIM THE GREAT WIS-DOM MAN-TRA, PRO-CLAIM THE
MAN-TRA LIKE THIS: GONE, GONE, GONE BE-YOND, GONE COM-
PLETE-LY BE-YOND, A-WAKEN-ING RIGHT NOW!

Some of Morihei's students learned *kototama* chanting at the Ichi-Kū-Kai
Dōjō in Tokyo and thus employ the *kototama*

TO-HO-KA-MI-E-MI-TA-ME

vigorously pronounced in conjunction with the ringing of a hand bell. This
chant was used in ancient divination ceremonies while a tortoise shell was
heated and cracked. Among other things, this *kototama* represents the establishment and maintenance of the physical world by the eight majestic deities,
and chanting it serves to integrate one's spirit with all elements of creation.

The above methods are based on classical forms, but as mentioned in chapter 2, any language can be used as a *kototama* to create other suitable chants.

Suggested Reading

As mentioned in the preface, *The Secrets of Aikidō* will be much more useful if the reader is familiar with the following books.

Abundant Peace, by John Stevens (Boston: Shambhala Publications, 1987), was the first full-length biography of Morihei in English. A revised and expanded version is *Invincible Warrior: An Illustrated Biography of Morihei Ueshiba* (Boston: Shambhala Publications, forthcoming).

Aikidō: The Way of Harmony, by John Stevens, under the direction of Rinjirō Shirata (Boston: Shambhala Publications, 1984), includes a brief biography of Morihei, outlines a good method of *chinkon-kishin* training, and contains much practical information about Aikidō.

The Art of Peace, by Morihei Ueshiba, translated by John Stevens (Boston: Shambhala Publications, 1992), contains Morihei's teachings adapted for a more general audience.

Budō: Teachings of the Founder of Aikidō, introduction by Kisshomaru Ueshiba, translation by John Stevens (Tokyo: Kodansha International, 1991), contains a brief biography of Morihei together with a translation of *Budō,* a teaching manual written by Morihei in 1938. There is also a series of photographs taken in the Noma Dōjō in 1936. A bilingual edition of *Budō Renshū,* an earlier, hand-drawn manual that first appeared in 1933, has been published by Minato Research, 20-13, Tadao 3 Chome, Machida-shi, Tokyo 194-02, Japan.

The Essence of Aikidō: Spiritual Teachings of Morihei Ueshiba, compiled by John Stevens (Tokyo: Kodansha International, 1993). *The Secrets of Aikidō* elaborates on and amplifies many of the teachings presented in *The Essence of Aikidō,* and the two books should be used in conjunction.

Kototama: The Secret Sounds of Aikidō, recorded by John Stevens, is available from *Aikido Today Magazine,* P.O. Box 1060, Claremont, CA 91711-1060 U.S.A. Telephone (909) 624-7770; U.S. customer order number 800-445-AIKI. A.T.M. can also supply most of the books mentioned here.

The Principles of Aikidō (1990) and *Aikidō and the Harmony of Na-*

ture (1993), two books by Mitsugi Saotome (Boston: Shambhala Publications), deal with the spiritual side of Aikidō from yet another perspective.

Shintō: At the Fountainhead of Japan, by J. Herbert (London: Allen & Unwin, 1967), is by far the best book on Shintō published in English. Unfortunately, it is long out of print, and copies may be found only in large libraries.

The Spirit of Aikidō, by Morihei's son, Kisshomaru Ueshiba (Tokyo: Kodansha International, 1984), discusses the inner factors of Aikidō from a traditional Japanese perspective.

Credits

Frontispiece, pp. 1, 8, 26, 32 (top), 33, 34, 37, 39, 40 (top), 46, 51, 59, 76, 84 (top & bottom), 85, 102, 105, 113 (left), 115, 116, 117 (top), 129, 137 courtesy of Kisshomaru Ueshiba; pp. 9 (top), 31 (right), 40 (bottom), 69, 80, 92, 93, 123, 124, 126, 127, 128, 131, 132, 134, 135, 138, 142 photography by Alan Nagahisa; pp. 9 (bottom), 10, 11, 12, 25 (top), 32 (bottom), 35 (right), 42, 43, 52, 58 (left), 60, 61, 67 (right), 71, 73 (left), 74, 75, 78, 79 (bottom), 84 (middle), 86, 94, 99, 100 (right), 107, 113 (right), 114, 118, 119, 121, 130, 136, 139, 140, 141 author's collection; pp. 13, 29, 41, 55, 56, 57, 67 (left), 68 (left), 72, 109, 120, 122, 125 courtesy of A. Nagahisa/W. von Krenner; pp. 83 (right), 103, 117 (bottom), 133 courtesy of Toma Rosenzweig; pp. 38, 50, 58 (right) the Gitter Collection, New Orleans; pp. 25 (bottom), 143 courtesy of K. Sunadomari; pp. 65, 66 photography by Tadashi Namba; p. 14 (left) private collection; p. 14 (right) Shinryū-Kai, the Netherlands; p. 21 (top) Archivio Opera di Santa Croce, Florence; p. 21 (bottom) private collection; p. 23 drawing by Colin Stevens; p. 30 from *Glauben, Wissen und Kunst der alten Hindus,* fig. 17; p. 31 (left) Zenshō-an Treasury, Tokyo; p. 35 (left) private collection; p. 47 Honolulu Academy of Arts, 1691.1, Gift of Robert Allerton, 1952; p. 48 Honolulu Academy of Arts, 1691.1 & 1692.1, Gift of John Gregg Allerton; p. 49 (top) calligraphy by Kijun Tokuyama; p. 49 (bottom) Tesshū-Kai, Tokyo; pp. 63, 64 Honolulu Academy of Arts, HAA 24, 449, Gift of James A. Michener; p. 68 (right) courtesy of the Fellowship of Reconciliation; p. 73 (right) Genshin Collection; p. 79 (top) Idemitsu Art Museum, Tokyo; p. 82 Zuigan-ji Treasury, Matsushima; p. 83 (left) Foreign Press Center, Kyodo; p. 89 (top) Collection: Robert Schaap, the Netherlands; p. 89 (bottom) Auchanbach Foundation for Graphic Art, 1963, 30.5559; p. 90 Copyright the British Museum; p. 91 Sendai City Museum; p. 97 courtesy of the Board of Trustees of the Victoria and Albert Museum; p. 98 the Cleveland Museum of Art, John L. Severance Fund 63.263; p. 100 (left) reprinted with the permission of Macmillian Publishing Company from *Erotic Spirituality* by Alan Watts, © 1971 by Alan Watts, illustrations by Eliot Elisofon © 1971 by Eliot Elisofon; p. 101 photo courtesy of Don Ed Hardy; p. 106 private collection.

We hope you enjoyed this title
from Echo Point Books & Media

Before Closing this Book, Two Good Things to Know

Buy Direct & Save

Go to www.echopointbooks.com (click "Our Titles" at top or click "For Echo Point Publishing" in the middle) to see our complete list of titles. We publish books on a wide variety of topics—from spirituality to auto repair.

Buy direct and save 10% at www.echopointbooks.com

DISCOUNT CODE: EPBUYER

Make Literary History and Earn $100 Plus Other Goodies Simply for Your Book Recommendation!

At Echo Point Books & Media we specialize in republishing out-of-print books that are united by one essential ingredient: high quality. Do you know of any great books that are no longer actively published? If so, please let us know. If we end up publishing your recommendation, you'll be adding a wee bit to literary culture and a bunch to our publishing efforts.

Here is how we will thank you:

- A free copy of the new version of your beloved book that includes acknowledgement of your skill as a sharp book scout.

- A free copy of another Echo Point title you like from echopointbooks.com.

- And, oh yes, we'll also send you a check for $100.

Since we publish an eclectic list of titles, we're interested in a wide range of books. So please don't be shy if you have obscure tastes or like books with a practical focus. To get a sense of what kind of books we publish, visit us at www.echopointbooks.com.

If you have a book that you think will work for us,
send us an email at editorial@echopointbooks.com

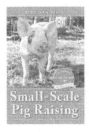
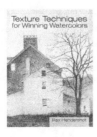
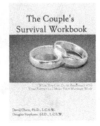
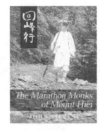
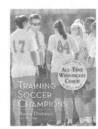